A SHORT HISTORY OF BRITISH MEDICAL ETHICS

ANDREAS-HOLGER MAEHLE

Ockham Publishing

Published in 2021 by Ockham Publishing in the United Kingdom

ISBN: 978-1-83919-083-4

Cover design by Claire Wood

www.ockham-publishing.com

Contents

Preface

In the context of current bioethics, the traditional ethics of doctors is often seen as dominated by etiquette and concern for professional interests rather than patient interests. In this short book I attempt to show that this assessment is wrong. Exploring medical ethics in Britain from the late eighteenth to the early twentieth century, i.e. the period in which the modern medical profession was formed, I illustrate how the doctors of this period faced difficult issues of medical practice. In making judgements about their options and actions, not only concerns about professional reputation but also about patients' welfare and the public good played an important role. I invite readers to make a brief tour with me through several key areas in the history of medical ethics to prove this point.

In the first chapter I discuss disciplinary actions of the General Medical Council, the regulatory body for medical practitioners in Britain, arguing that we can learn about ethical standards of the profession by analysing how it dealt with cases of (alleged) misconduct. Studying a range of controversial behaviours, from matters of personal and sexual conduct to professional issues such as medical advertising and the 'covering' of unqualified assistants, I demonstrate that the protection of patients and of a wider public interest in responsible medical practice were essential considerations in the GMC's disciplinary proceedings. Chapter 2 focuses on nineteenth-century doctor–patient relations, especially the questions to what extent doctors sought their patients' consent to treatments and how well patients were informed by their medical attendants. I do this through the discussion of a legal case from the 1890s, in which a doctor was accused by his patient of having removed her ovaries without valid consent. Issues of gender, professional ethics, and law, as well as the historical development of gynaecological surgery, came into this particular case, but in more general terms I describe how doctors' paternalistic attitudes and their tradition of restricted truth-telling in the patient's presumed interest had become a problem by the turn of the twentieth century.

Widening the perspective again, I review in the third chapter the key works of British medical ethics from the 1770s to the early 1900s, so that readers can appreciate what the authors of this period themselves thought to be the most important ethical issues and what conceptions of a good medical practitioner they developed. The relationships between professional subgroups, i.e. between physicians, surgeons, and apothecaries, and later between specialist consultants and general practitioners, took much space here, but so did a broad range of patient-related matters, including compassion, confidentiality, mutual trust and obligations, clinical experimentation, and doctors' continuing duty to the dying and their families. In the fourth and fifth chapters, I turn to situations in which nineteenth-century medical practitioners had to make hard moral choices. Chapter 4 examines how they dealt with desperate cases of severely obstructed labour where the baby could neither be delivered manually nor by using the forceps. Practitioners then had to decide whether they should sacrifice the life of the unborn child through craniotomy in the hope of saving the mother, or risk the woman's life in daring to perform a Caesarean section, which then had a very high mortality rate. Other moral choices, discussed in chapter 5, concerned confidentiality in cases of illegal abortion and venereal diseases. Here I show how doctors grappled with the question of disclosure without the patient's consent in the interest of the public or a third party. They had to balance their commitment to the individual patient, which called for strict confidentiality, with wider legal and social expectations of their role, which might include reporting a case of criminal abortion to the police, especially if the woman was dying from the intervention, or warning contact persons of patients infected with a venereal disease. I also discuss here doctors' situations as witnesses in court when they were required to reveal private information about their patients.

History of medical ethics involves not just analysing past problems but also giving voice to the authors of the time and re-thinking practitioners' controversial cases. It is in this way that we can begin to perceive in fairness past doctors' conduct and ethical choices. I hope that readers will find this exploration an exciting subject as well as helpful in gaining a historical perspective on doctors' ethics.

Andreas-Holger Maehle
Durham University, September 2019

Chapter 1

Medical Ethics and the General Medical Council

Introduction[1]

Medical ethics in Britain during the long nineteenth century tends to have a bad name among scholars. Jeffrey Berlant and Ivan Waddington have claimed that doctors' ethics in that period were self-serving, aiming more at supporting the interests of the profession than at protecting patients. In particular they have suggested that regular doctors used ethics as a strategy to demarcate themselves from unlicensed and unorthodox practitioners and as an instrument to mitigate competition within their profession by focusing on rules for maintaining smooth intra-professional relationships between physicians, surgeons and apothecaries, and between consultants and general practitioners. Furthermore, medical ethics was characterised as a trust-inducing

---

[1] This chapter is based on my article, Andreas-Holger Maehle, 'Beyond Professional Self-interest: Medical Ethics and the Disciplinary Function of the General Medical Council of the United Kingdom, 1858-1914', *Social History of Medicine*, 2018, doi: 10.1093/shm/hky072, vol. 33/1 (2020), pp. 41-56.

device vis-à-vis the public and as a tool for monopolisation of the healthcare market.[2] In addition, bioethicists Laurence McCullough and Robert Veatch have suggested that after promising beginnings in the late eighteenth century, British medical ethics lost its way: while the well-known lectures of Edinburgh professor of medicine John Gregory on the duties and qualifications of a physician of 1772 had been influenced by contemporary Scottish Common Sense philosophy, so the argument goes, subsequent writers on medical ethics got too much embroiled in intra-professional issues and lost the connection with moral philosophy.[3]

Only occasionally this negative picture of medical ethics in the long nineteenth century has been qualified in some respects. For example, reinterpreting Thomas Percival's influential text *Medical Ethics* of 1803, which had been blamed,

---

[2] Jeffrey Lionel Berlant, *Profession and Monopoly: A Study of Medicine in the United States and Great Britain* (Berkeley, University of California Press, 1975), pp. 68-81; Ivan Waddington, 'The Development of Medical Ethics – A Sociological Analysis', *Medical History* 19 (1975), pp. 36-51; idem, *The Medical Profession in the Industrial Revolution* (Dublin, Gill and Macmillan, 1984), pp. 153-175. See also Anne Digby, *Making a Medical Living: Doctors and Patients in the English Market for Medicine, 1720-1911* (Cambridge, Cambridge University Press, 1994), pp. 59-62.

[3] John Gregory, *Lectures on the Duties and Qualifications of a Physician* (London, W. Strahan and T. Cadell, 1772); Laurence B. McCullough, *John Gregory and the Invention of Professional Medical Ethics and the Profession of Medicine* (Dordrecht, Kluwer Academic Publishers, 1998); Robert M. Veatch, *Disrupted Dialogue: Medical Ethics and the Collapse of Physician-Humanist Communication (1770-1980)* (New York, Oxford University Press, 2005). See also Lisbeth Haakonssen, *Medicine and Morals in the Enlightenment: John Gregory, Thomas Percival and Benjamin Rush* (Amsterdam, Rodopi, 1997).

since Chauncey Leake's edition of 1927, for having promoted an intra-professional focus over attention to doctor–patient relations, Robert Baker has identified elements in it that seem to reflect contemporary social contract theory.[4] Duncan Wilson has recently highlighted English physician Jukes Styrap, author of a late nineteenth-century code of medical ethics, as an example of a writer who emphasised a link between professional and public interest by arguing that patients were best served by trusting a unified medical profession that was clearly distinct from 'tradesmen and quacks'.[5] Similarly, Andrew Morrice found that doctors involved in the ethical work of the British Medical Association

[4] Robert Baker, 'Deciphering Percival's Code', in idem, Dorothy Porter and Roy Porter (eds), *The Codification of Medical Morality*, vol. 1: *Medical Ethics and Etiquette in the Eighteenth Century* (Dordrecht, Kluwer Academic Publishers, 1993), pp. 179-211; Thomas Percival, 'Medical Ethics: Or, A Code of Institutes and Precepts, Adapted to the Professional Conduct of Physicians and Surgeons' (1803), in C. D. Leake (ed.), *Percival's Medical Ethics* (Huntington, NY, Robert E. Krieger Publishing Company, 1975), pp. 61-205. See also Gary S. Belkin, 'History and bioethics: The uses of Thomas Percival', *Medical Humanities Review* 12 (1998), pp. 39-59, who gives a variety of interpretations of Percival as learned gentleman, philosopher, and political actor.

[5] Duncan Wilson, *The Making of British Bioethics* (Manchester, Manchester University Press, 2014), p. 29; Jukes Styrap, *A Code of Medical Ethics: With Remarks on the Duties of Practitioners to their Patients, and the Obligations of Patients to their Medical Advisers: also on the Duties of the Profession to the Public, and the Obligations of the Public to the Faculty* (London, J. & A. Churchill, 1878). See also Peter Bartrip, 'An Introduction to Jukes Styrap's *A Code of Medical Ethics* (1878)', in Robert Baker (ed.), *The Codification of Medical Morality*, vol. 2: *Anglo-American Medical Ethics and Medical Jurisprudence in the Nineteenth Century* (Dordrecht, Kluwer Academic Publishers, 1995), pp. 145-148.

during the early twentieth century described professional interests and public interests as interlinked.[6]

Moreover, Roger Cooter has suggested that one should not adopt unreservedly Berlant's and Waddington's characterisations of the historical medical profession, because at the time of their writing, in the 1970s and early 1980s, the emergence of an apparently lay-driven bioethics would have stimulated them to focus on, and criticize, the self-interested features of the professional ethics of medical men.[7] Historical accounts of the rise of bioethics during the second half of the twentieth century, especially by the field's pioneers, have indeed emphasised the role of non-medical protagonists, such as theologians, philosophers and lawyers, who were keen to put patient and public interests into the foreground of debates on ethics in medicine.[8] Bioethicists who wished to demarcate the 'old' medical ethics from their

[6] Andrew A. G. Morrice, '"Honour and Interests": Medical Ethics and the British Medical Association', in Andreas-Holger Maehle and Johanna Geyer-Kordesch (eds), *Historical and Philosophical Perspectives on Biomedical Ethics: From Paternalism to Autonomy?* (Aldershot, Ashgate, 2002), pp. 11-35, on p. 15.

[7] Roger Cooter with Claudia Stein, *Writing History in the Age of Biomedicine* (New Haven and London, Yale University Press, 2013), p. 175.

[8] Albert R. Jonsen, *The Birth of Bioethics* (New York and Oxford, Oxford University Press, 1998); Daniel Callahan, *In Search of the Good: A Life in Bioethics* (Cambridge, Mass. and London, MIT Press, 2012); David J. Rothman, *Strangers at the Bedside: A History of How Law and Bioethics Transformed Medical Decision Making* (BasicBooks USA, 1991).

'new' interdisciplinary ethics may have unwittingly distorted historical perspectives by paying too little attention to the patient-related aspects of doctors' traditional ethics.[9]

Going beyond these qualifications and criticisms of the traditional view of nineteenth-century medical ethics, I seek to further challenge it by looking, in this chapter, into evidence for the contemporary practice of medical ethics (rather than just its normative texts) within a state-authorised system for the control of doctors' conduct in the United Kingdom.[10] To what extent did nineteenth-century medical ethics, as a practice, support interests of patients and the public at large? What was the relationship between professional interests and patients' interests? My focus here is the disciplinary function of the General Council of Medical Education and Registration (nowadays known as the General Medical Council or GMC), which was established through an Act of Parliament in 1858. As historian Michael Roberts has shown in his analysis of the genesis of this Act, three major factors contributed to this piece of medical reform: a drive towards professional representation from the rising

---

[9] For a critical assessment of the rise of bioethics and the 'bioethicists' tale' see Roger Cooter, 'The Ethical Body', in idem and John Pickstone (eds), *Companion to Medicine in the Twentieth Century* (London and New York, Routledge, 2003), pp. 451-468. See also Gary S. Belkin, 'Moving Beyond Bioethics: history and the search for medical humanism', *Perspectives in Biology and Medicine* 47 (2004), pp. 372-385.

[10] For discussion of the medical ethics literature of the nineteenth century, see chapter 3, below.

group of general practitioners at a time when the old tripartite structure distinguishing physicians, surgeons and apothecaries was becoming dysfunctional; a public interest in ensuring competency and honourable behaviour of medical practitioners, a task which traditionally lay in the hands of the medical corporations (royal colleges); and the state's interest in qualified medical service in public health and in the workhouses for the able-bodied poor which had been established with the Poor Law Amendment Act 1834.[11] Besides its role in monitoring standards of medical education, the General Council was given the task to maintain a Register of practitioners holding officially recognised medical qualifications. As a corollary to this latter function the Council was authorised to erase the names of those from the Register who had been wrongly placed on it; who had been convicted by a court of a misdemeanour (offence) or felony (crime); or who had been found guilty by the Council of 'infamous conduct in any professional respect'.[12] Drawing upon the *Minutes of the General Council of Medical Education and Registration* for the years 1859 to 1914, I argue that the

---

[11] Michael J. D. Roberts, 'The Politics of Professionalization: MPs, Medical Men, and the 1858 Medical Act', *Medical History* 53 (2009), pp. 37-56.
[12] Walter Pyke-Lees, *Centenary of the General Medical Council 1858-1958: The History and Present Work of the Council* (London, William Clowes & Sons, [1958]), pp. 1-4.

disciplinary cases can give us a clue to contemporary standards of medical professional ethics.[13]

During this period the GMC dealt with over 400 such cases.[14] Legal and quantitative analysis of the GMC's cases from 1859 up to 1990 by Russell G. Smith has led to the criticism that the Council sometimes disciplined medical practitioners before giving them specific ethical guidance on the issue concerned.[15] However, the disciplinary cases, when read in greater detail and in their specific contexts, do reveal the 'ethical compass' of the Council's physicians and surgeons who had been invested with the state's authority to decide on the professional fate of other medical practitioners. Referring to a variety of cases, ranging from fraudulent registration, sexual misconduct, and breach of confidence to alleged negligence in post-mortem examination, covering of unqualified assistants, and advertising, I suggest that the

---

[13] *Minutes of the General Council of Medical Education and Registration of the United Kingdom* (London, W. J. & S. Golbourn, 1863ff). Hereafter cited as *Minutes*.

[14] Russell G. Smith, *Medical Discipline: The Professional Conduct Jurisdiction of the General Medical Council, 1858-1990* (Oxford, Clarendon Press, 1994), pp. 238-255.

[15] Ibid., 57, 70; R. G. Smith, 'The Development of Ethical Guidance for Medical Practitioners by the General Medical Council', *Medical History* 37 (1993), pp. 56-67, on p. 63; R. G. Smith, 'Legal Precedent and Medical Ethics: Some Problems Encountered by the General Medical Council in Relying upon Precedent when Declaring Acceptable Standards of Professional Conduct', in Robert Baker (ed.), *The Codification of Medical Morality*, vol. 2: *Anglo-American Medical Ethics and Medical Jurisprudence in the Nineteenth Century* (Dordrecht, Kluwer Academic Publishers, 1995), pp. 205-218, on p. 212.

medical men of the General Council tried to implement values that lay in patients' as well as doctors' interests.

The General Medical Council and its Register

Before going into specific cases, we need to clarify who the members of the GMC were that sat in judgement over their colleagues. Initially, the Council comprised twenty-four members: nine represented the medical Royal Colleges of London, Edinburgh, Glasgow and Dublin, the Society of Apothecaries in London, and the Apothecaries' Hall in Dublin; seven represented the four English and three Irish universities and two the four Scottish universities; and six were nominated by the Queen on the advice of her Privy Council. All members were medically qualified men and can be seen as representing the professional establishment of the time.[16] Only after a new Medical Act in 1886, five additional members were directly elected by the registered medical practitioners of the United Kingdom, a step which reflected the increased importance of general practice at that time.[17] It also then became a requirement for registration that practitioners had certified proficiency in all the three main branches, 'medicine, surgery and midwifery', rather

---

[16] Pyke-Lees, *Centenary*, p. 3; Anne Digby, *The Evolution of General Practice 1850–1948* (Oxford and New York, Oxford University Press, 1999), p. 39.
[17] Donald MacAlister, 'The General Medical Council: Its Powers and Its Work', *British Medical Journal* 1906, 2 (2388), pp. 817-23, p. 820.

than just in medicine and/or surgery.[18] In the period that I am looking at, 1858 to 1914, the General Medical Council had nine Presidents – eminent physicians or surgeons, from Sir Benjamin Brodie (term of office 1858–1860) to Sir Donald MacAlister (term of office 1904–1931).[19] By the early twentieth century, the Crown and the universities could appoint laymen to the Council, but did not choose to do so until 1926. From the 1880s, however, it became customary that the Council's solicitor and a barrister, as Legal Assessor, were present during disciplinary proceedings, and the accused medical practitioners also brought (or sent) their defence lawyers. The disciplinary proceedings thus adopted a format that was similar to court proceedings.[20] Britain was not alone in institutionalising medical discipline in this quasi-legal manner; Prussia, for example, legally introduced so-called medical courts of honour for this purpose in 1899.[21]

---

[18] Roberts, 'Politics of Professionalization', p. 53.

[19] Pyke-Lees, *Centenary*, p. 30. Brodie had demonstrated his interest in medical professional ethics long before his appointment as President of the General Council, see Benjamin Brodie, 'Introductory Discourse on the Duties and Conduct of Medical Students and Practitioners. Addressed to the Students of St. George's Hospital, October 2, 1843', in *The Works of Sir Benjamin Collins Brodie*, collected and arranged by Charles Hawkins, 3 vols (London, Longman, Green etc., 1865), vol. 1, pp. 485-505.

[20] MacAlister, 'General Medical Council', p. 820; Smith, 'Legal Precedent', p. 207.

[21] See Andreas-Holger Maehle, *Doctors, Honour and the Law: Medical Ethics in Imperial Germany* (Basingstoke, Palgrave Macmillan, 2009), pp. 6-46.

The preamble of the 1858 Medical Act stated that its purpose was to enable 'persons requiring medical aid [...] to distinguish qualified from unqualified practitioners'.[22] That was in essence the function of the Medical Register, on which only those practitioners who held a recognised qualification from one of the above-mentioned licensing institutions represented on the Council, or who had been practising medicine in 1815 were admitted. In 1859, almost 15,000 names were on this register, and the number increased to about 23,000 by 1880, and c. 50,000 by 1924.[23] Being unregistered, however, did not prevent someone from practising medicine. Registration was only required for fulfilling official functions, such as issuing a death certificate, or for holding positions in public employment, e.g. serving as a medical officer or practising under the 1911 National Health Insurance scheme. Also, only registered practitioners were entitled to sue in the courts for their fees.[24] Nevertheless, the prestige and professional legitimacy that registration brought are not only reflected in the rising numbers of registered practitioners but also in disciplinary cases in

[22] Cited in MacAlister, 'General Medical Council', p. 817.

[23] Pyke-Lees, *Centenary*, p. 3. According to Digby an important reason for the increase in the numbers of registered practitioners was the growing number of graduate entrants in the Register; by 1913 the total number of practitioners on the Register had reached about 42,000. Cf. Digby, *Making a Medical Living*, pp. 15-16.

[24] MacAlister, 'General Medical Council', p. 817; Margaret Stacey, *Regulating British Medicine: The General Medical Council* (Chichester, John Wiley & Sons, 1992), pp. 18-19; Roberts, 'Politics of Professionalization', p. 47.

which practitioners erased from the Register keenly sought to have their names restored. For example, Leeds doctor Henry Arthur Allbutt, who had been struck off in 1887 for publishing a booklet including contraceptive advice which was considered detrimental to 'public morals', took the General Council to court to have his name placed back on the Register and to seek damages for libel.[25] Other practitioners wrote to the Council with long apologies or detailed justifications of the conduct that had led to erasure of their names, hoping to have them restored.[26]

Examples of Disciplinary Cases and their Interpretation

It is therefore unsurprising that a series of early disciplinary cases were concerned with fraudulent registration, i.e. with practitioners who falsely declared to have a registrable

---

[25] *Minutes*, vol. 24, 1887, pp. 122-123, 307-313, 316-317; vol. 26, 1889, 181-183. The publication concerned was Arthur H. Albutt, *The Wife's Handbook: How a woman should order herself during Pregnancy, in the Lying-in Room, and after Delivery*, 2nd edn (London, W. J. Ramsey, 1886). Chapter VII (pp. 46-50) gave details of various contraceptive techniques and devices, including the names of the firms from where to obtain the latter. Advertisements for the devices, such as 'The Improved Check Pessary' and 'Malthusian Appliance – The Improved Vertical and Reverse Syringe', appeared at the end of the booklet. For further details and the neo-Malthusian context of the Allbutt case see Angus McLaren, *Birth Control in Nineteenth-Century England* (New York, Holmes & Meier Publishers, 1978), pp. 112, 132-133.

[26] See e.g. *Minutes*, vol. 19, 1882, pp. 83-85 (following erasure in 1877 because of criminal conviction for attempted sodomy); vol. 33, 1896, pp. 232-237 (following erasure in 1894 for advertising for a company). On the latter case (Herbert Tibbits), see below.

qualification or tried to obtain one by fraud. If the Council found practitioners guilty of such an offence, they were erased from the Register.[27] While these decisions were recorded without much comment one can safely assume that the Council aimed to fulfil here its task of enabling the public to identify qualified practitioners. One might, of course, also take the more sceptical line of interpreting those erasures as a process of professional boundary demarcation from the 'unqualified', carried out in the economic interest of the 'qualified' practitioners. The issue of fraud in medical titles was as such not new: already in the early 1850s there had been complaints about this matter in connection with the publication of the (unofficial) British Medical Directory.[28]

It would be rash, however, to view the early disciplinary cases simply as expressions of professional self-interest. In 1873, for example, the Council erased a medical doctor from the Register because of sexual relations with a female patient. The initial complaint, that he had 'seduced and carnally known' her, had been made by the patient's uncle, a solicitor.[29] The doctor's petition, two years later, to have his name restored to the Register was rejected, as was his further request to this effect in the following year.[30] Only at the

---

[27] See e.g. *Minutes*, vol. 1, 1863, pp. 94-97, 103-104, 213, 245, 251; vol. 2, 1864, 341-342

[28] 'Fictitious Medical Titles', *The Lancet*, August, 21, 1852, p. 179.

[29] *Minutes*, vol. 10, 1872-73, pp. 149-150.

[30] *Minutes*, vol. 12, 1875, p. 23; vol. 13, 1876, p. 333.

third attempt, after a total of eleven years, was his named restored.[31] This was a typical case of 'infamous conduct in a professional respect' that constituted a violation of moral standards of the medical profession in relation to patients. The rule against sexual relations with patients had already been part of the Hippocratic Oath.[32] It was also behind the vow to practise 'chastely' in Edinburgh University's Medical Oath, which had been sworn since the early 1730s.[33] In the moralistic climate of the nineteenth century the rule aimed both at protecting patients and at preventing reputational damage to the profession.[34] Seen in this light it is understandable that the GMC in this disciplinary case repeatedly rejected the doctor's application to restore his name to the Register – taking a firm line in a matter like this protected the GMC's own reputation.

Another early GMC case concerned medical confidentiality – a rule likewise mentioned in the Hippocratic Oath, but also in nineteenth-century British works on medical deontology, such as Percival's *Medical Ethics* and Michael

---

[31] Smith, *Medical Discipline*, p. 240.

[32] 'Into as many houses as I may enter, I will go for the benefit of the ill, while being far from all voluntary and destructive injustice, especially from sexual acts, both upon women's bodies and upon men's, both of the free and of the slaves.' See Steven H. Miles, *The Hippocratic Oath and the Ethics of Medicine* (New York, Oxford University Press, 2004), pp. xiv, 139-148.

[33] Robert Baker, *Before Bioethics: A History of American Medical Ethics from the Colonial Period to the Bioethics Revolution* (New York, Oxford University Press, 2013), pp. 37, 49.

[34] See also Digby, *Evolution of British General Practice*, p. 282.

Ryan's *A Manual of Medical Jurisprudence*.[35] This case concerned a medical doctor, John Pattison, who had qualified in New York but was practising in London. In 1868, he had accused the husband of a patient with breast cancer of 'stubbornness', because he had refused to follow the doctor's advice to take her after local treatment of the tumour for recuperation to the south of France over the winter months. Instead, the husband eventually took her at the end of January to the seaside at Hastings, where she died a few days later. The doctor was further aggrieved by the fact that the husband refused to pay the full bill for numerous home visits to the sick wife, and he warned the husband in writing that he was going to publish the circumstances and details of the case in a medical book.[36] When the husband returned the doctor's letters, which included accusations of 'shabby conduct', to the dead letter office, Pattison sent them by open post, so that they could be read by anyone, and threatened that he would next time write them on cardboard and send them to the husband's club. The husband, Charles Hay Frewen, a Royal sheriff and former Member of Parliament,

---

[35] 'And about whatever I may see or hear in treatment, or even without treatment, in the life of human beings – things that should not ever be blurted out outside – I will remain silent, holding such things to be unutterable.' See Miles, *Hippocratic Oath*, pp. xiv, 149-157. Percival, 'Medical Ethics', p. 90; Michael Ryan, 'A Manual of Medical Jurisprudence and State Medicine' (1836), in H. Brody, Z. Meghani and K. Greenwald (eds), *Michael Ryan's Writings on Medical Ethics* (Dordrecht, Springer, 2010), pp. 79-222, on pp. 157-158.
[36] *Minutes*, vol. 7, 1869, pp. 41-45.

took the doctor to court for libel and breach of the peace.[37] At the second court hearing Pattison apologised through his lawyer to Frewen and assured to have his book published without including the case history concerned. Frewen's lawyer then withdrew the charges, so that the court, somewhat reluctantly, dismissed the case.[38] However, the General Medical Council, on learning about this court case from newspaper reports, decided to hold its own inquiry into the matter, found Pattison guilty of infamous conduct in a professional respect and erased his name in 1869 from the Register. His petition in 1871 to have his name restored was rejected by the Council.[39] The sparse GMC Minutes unfortunately give us no information about the Council's reasoning behind their decisions. However, it is clear that the deontological literature, in particular Percival and Ryan, had described unauthorised disclosures as unethical. As Ryan had put it in 1836:

> The confidence reposed in him [i.e. the medical practitioner], and revelations made to him, during his professional attendance, are such that honour commands him not to abuse the one, or publish the other, unless in our courts of justice, which have the power to compel him.

---

[37] 'Court of Queen's Bench, Westminster, Jan. 25', *The Times*, issue 26344, January 26, 1869, p. 11.
[38] 'Court of Queen's Bench, Westminster, Feb. 1', *The Times*, issue 26350, February 2, 1869, pp. 8-9.
[39] *Minutes*, vol. 7, 1869, pp. 41-45, 159, 162; vol. 9, 1871, p. 14.

[...] such secrets are not to be divulged without the greatest necessity [...].[40]

Russell Smith has identified Pattison's case as the GMC's first disciplinary case on medical confidentiality, and deplores that the GMC began to publish guidance on this topic only over a hundred years later.[41] However, it is quite clear from the context of the case that the Council acted on a contemporary, professional as well as public expectation about the requirements of discreet behaviour in a doctor and enforced this social expectation through its decisions. In 1851, the Scottish Court of Sessions case of A.B. v. C.D., in which a doctor was accused of having disclosed sensitive family information of the plaintiff to the minister of his parish, had established that the relationship between medical adviser and the person consulting him implied an obligation of secrecy that, if violated, could give proper grounds for legal action. Only in a court of law doctors were expected, and compelled, to testify concerning patient details.[42]

---

[40] Ryan, 'Manual', p. 157.

[41] Smith, 'Legal Precedent', p. 211. Actually, GMC Legal Assessor Muir Mackenzie prepared a memorandum on the obligations of medical practitioners regarding professional secrecy in 1899 which was published in the *British Medical Journal* and *The Lancet*. Cf. Angus H. Ferguson, *Should a Doctor Tell? The Evolution of Medical Confidentiality in Britain* (Farnham, Ashgate, 2013), pp. 28, 37-38; Andreas-Holger Maehle, *Contesting Medical Confidentiality: Origins of the Debate in the United States, Britain, and Germany* (Chicago and London, University of Chicago Press, 2016), p. 30.

[42] Walter F. Pratt, *Privacy in Britain* (Lewisburg, Bucknell University Press, and London, Associated University Presses, 1979), pp. 46-47; Ferguson, *Should a Doctor Tell?*, pp. 24-26; and Maehle, *Contesting Medical Confidentiality*, pp. 9-10.

In Pattison's case, then, the GMC acted on the supposed interests of the patient and her husband's demand of medical secrecy. These interests were apparently not in conflict with professional interests which were concerned about the public reputation of medical practitioners.

Another case indicated, however, the limits of the GMC's disciplinary role. In April 1881, the King and Queen's College of Physicians in Ireland sent a complaint about Richard Albert Shipman Prosser, a Member of the Royal College of Surgeons of England and Licentiate of the Society of Apothecaries in London, to the General Medical Council. Prosser had sworn in a coroner's court that he had performed a post-mortem examination on a female patient's body, in which he examined the kidneys and all other abdominal viscera, and found the kidneys healthy. On the basis of this examination, he had accused the medical practitioner who had treated the patient of having caused her death by negligence. On this evidence the practitioner concerned, Edward Hyacinth O'Leary, a Licentiate of the King and Queen's College of Physicians, had been charged with manslaughter and imprisoned. A second post-mortem examination by two other medical practitioners then showed, however, that the kidneys had not been removed from their place during the autopsy and that the other abdominal organs also appeared to have been incompletely examined. Following this information the manslaughter charge against O'Leary was dropped, and he was released from prison.

King and Queen's College held that Prosser's behaviour amounted to infamous conduct in a professional respect and asked the GMC to erase his name from the Register.[43] So in this case, Prosser, who had made the accusation of negligence about a fellow-practitioner, was himself suspected of having been negligent, namely in his post-mortem examination, with the serious consequence that the practitioner accused by him had been indicted with manslaughter and arrested.[44]

The initial response of the GMC Branch Council for England, which first looked at the complaint, was that this case did not seem to be one in which the Council could 'usefully take action'. King and Queen's College, dissatisfied with this reply, repeated its complaint in May 1881. The Branch Council was still unwilling to take the matter further, seeing it as a case of 'conflicting evidence' and noting that no legal action had been taken against Prosser for perjury. However, the central General Medical Council decided that the Branch Council should inquire further into Prosser's conduct in this case.[45] Having obtained and considered their solicitor's report on the case and having consulted with the General

---

[43] *Minutes*, vol. 18, 1881, pp. 266-267.

[44] On nineteenth-century notions of negligence see Kim Price, *Medical Negligence in Victorian Britain: The Crisis of Care under the English Poor Law, c. 1834-1900* (London, Bloomsbury Academic, 2015).

[45] *Minutes*, vol. 18, 1881, pp. 213-214, 267; vol. 19, 1882, pp. 100, 197-199, 212.

Council's solicitor, the Branch Council concluded eventually, in March 1883, nearly two years after the initial complaint, that there were no grounds for finding Prosser guilty of infamous conduct in a professional respect.[46] In spite of the intervention of two GMC members, who wanted to see the report of the second post-mortem examination, the General Medical Council agreed with this conclusion the following month.[47]

Apart from throwing a light on the power relations between a royal college, the General Medical Council and one of its branch councils, the Prosser case illustrates the difficulties the GMC had early on in forming an opinion on the quality of medical performance. The reference to 'conflicting evidence' is quite revealing in this regard. In the end, the GMC followed the legal assessments of its solicitors, which in turn were informed by the decisions of the general courts involved. It summoned neither Prosser nor O'Leary to hear them directly about their sides of the case, whereas it had summoned the accused practitioners in the sexual misconduct and breach of confidentiality cases mentioned above. So how did the early GMC then address its task of protecting the public against poorly performing medical practitioners, as distinct from practitioners whose moral conduct was questionable?

---

[46] *Minutes*, vol. 20, 1883, pp. 222-223.
[47] *Minutes*, vol. 20, 1883, pp. 32-33.

Two Major Issues: Covering Unqualified Assistants and Medical Advertising

As the mentioned cases on fraudulent registration indicate, the GMC's approach focused on medical qualifications, and in fact the related matter of covering unqualified assistants became a key issue in the late nineteenth century. The problem was, in short, that some qualified medical men, who ran large practices, employed unqualified assistants (that is, assistants without a registrable qualification) and allowed them to do unsupervised work which was supposed only to be carried out by a qualified medical practitioner. Such assistants sometimes gave the wrong impression to patients that they were regular doctors.[48] A GMC Committee looking into substantial evidence on this issue concluded in 1883 that the system of employing unqualified assistants was widespread in England and Wales, especially in general practice for the large mining and manufacturing populations. The Committee expressed concern that this system was blocking employment opportunities and earnings for qualified assistants. But above all it saw the system as 'fraud on the public', comparable to the public offence of lawyers who covered persons falsely pretending to be a solicitor or attorney, which was punishable with withdrawal of the lawyer's practising license and a prison sentence for the unqualified person. The qualified medical practitioners who

[48] *Minutes*, vol. 21, 1884, p. 252; vol. 23, 1886, p. 117.

covered an unqualified assistant, for example by signing medical or death certificates on patients they had not seen themselves, were held to be guilty of 'infamous conduct'. Their behaviour frustrated the fundamental principle of the 1858 Medical Act that it should enable the public to distinguish between qualified and unqualified practitioners.[49] So, in this matter the GMC aimed to protect the public against incompetent treatment, though not by control of performance but indirectly by control of medical employment. It acted here in the interest of the public, while simultaneously supporting the employment opportunities for junior qualified practitioners.

The Committee's recommendation to discipline practitioners who covered unqualified assistants was adopted by the GMC, which decided to publish a warning on this issue in the same year, 1883.[50] This was the first of the GMC's official Warning Notices, which specified types of behaviour that might lead to a disciplinary inquiry and erasure from the Register.[51] Numerous charges of covering unqualified assistants were heard by the GMC until this type of disciplinary offence became less frequent in the years after 1900.[52] A particularly prominent case of this kind was that of Dr

---

[49] *Minutes*, vol. 20, 1883, pp. 39-45, 51-85.
[50] *Minutes*, vol. 20, 1883, p. 91.
[51] By 1914 Warning Notices had also been issued regarding issues with certification, sale of poisons, dangerous drugs, association with unqualified practitioners, and advertising and canvassing. Smith, 'Development of Ethical Guidance', p. 61.
[52] Smith, *Medical Discipline*, pp. 103, 241-255.

Walter Day and Mr William Davenport in 1886. It had been reported by the Deputy Coroner for Westminster, Athelstan Braxton Hicks, to the Secretary of State for the Home Department, before the latter forwarded the material to the GMC, asking the Council to deal with it 'as the practice of employing unqualified practitioners as assistants by medical men is very common, especially by medical men presiding over dispensaries'.[53] A coroner's inquest had been held over the body of a 53-year-old labourer, as Dr John Pugh, who had been called by the family for emergency help on the night the man was dying, suspected that the patient had only been treated in his last illness by an unqualified practitioner, Davenport, who worked as an assistant in Dr Day's dispensary. Pugh had therefore refused to give a death certificate and written to the Registrar of Deaths. Dr Day had subsequently signed the death certificate, wrongly entering as the last date he had seen the patient the day on which Davenport had actually attended him. However, Day claimed to have personally seen to the patient in the dispensary two days earlier when the latter had presented with symptoms of acute bronchitis. While the post-mortem examination did not reveal anything suspicious, indicating heart failure upon congestion of the lungs, and Davenport's treatment appeared to have been appropriate, the coroner

[53] *Minutes*, vol. 23, 1886, p. 114.

was alarmed about the circumstances of the death certificate, in particular as Davenport had a previous conviction for perjury. Concerned about 'the poor' being treated by unqualified men who were unable to give valid certificates for their insurance clubs, Braxton Hicks had informed the Home Secretary. The latter had subsequently consulted the Registrar-General, who advised against taking legal action against Dr Day, given that he had declared under oath to have personally seen the patient only two days before the patient's death.[54] Braxton Hicks' involvement as coroner and the holding of an inquest over the patient's body was in line with a general, though not uncontroversial policy at this time: that all deaths not certified by a registered medical practitioner should be referred to the coroner, who would then decide whether an inquest should be held.[55] As Ian Burney has argued, the threat to a deceased person's family of the unwanted publicity of a coroner's inquest can be seen as an instrument of the medical profession to discipline the population into seeking qualified medical care and avoiding unlicensed practitioners.[56] While this interpretation points to professional self-interest in cases such as this, there appears to have also been genuine concern about the quality

[54] *Minutes*, vol. 23, 1886, pp. 114-121.

[55] Ian A. Burney, *Bodies of Evidence: Medicine and the Politics of the English Inquest 1830-1926* (Baltimore and London, Johns Hopkins University Press, 2000), pp. 75-76.

[56] Ibid., p. 77.

of care provided by unqualified assistants such as Davenport. The General Medical Council, upon advice of its solicitor, decided to take no action against Dr Day, but took the opportunity to inform the Home Department and the Privy Council about the recent GMC inquiry into the issue of employing unqualified assistants, including the subsequent Warning Notice of 1883 and a resolution then taken to ask for legislation on the matter.[57] It also defined more clearly the circumstances under which a registered practitioner might be 'censured' for covering an unqualified assistant. This was held to be likely if the unqualified assistant practised 'in complete substitution' for the registered practitioner's services or under circumstances where 'due personal supervision and control' by the latter were not, or could not be, exercised.[58]

The implications of this position of the GMC are illustrated by another disciplinary case on covering an unqualified assistant, in 1910. Being the first case in which the British Medical Association acted as official complainant to the GMC, it received detailed coverage in the *British Medical Journal*.[59] As the BMA's Medical Secretary, James Smith

[57] *Minutes*, vol. 23, 1886, p. 256; vol. 24, 1887, pp. 143-144, 357.

[58] *Minutes*, vol. 25, 1888, pp. 36-37.

[59] 'Disciplinary Cases before the Medical Council', *British Medical Journal*, June 4, 1910, 1366-1367; General Council of Medical Education and Registration, 'Medical Disciplinary Cases. The Case of Mr. David Thomas Jones', *Supplement to the British Medical Journal*, June 4, 1910, pp. 340-347. The BMA had a Central Ethical Committee since 1902. See Morrice, 'Medical Ethics and the British Medical Association'.

Whitaker, asserted in the relevant GMC hearing 'the case was of considerable public importance'.[60] David Thomas Jones, a qualified surgeon running a large practice with three partners in Sheffield, stood accused of having allowed his medically unqualified dispenser and surgery attendant, William Perry, to attend one of his working-class patients, Mrs Alice Hannah Nicholson, when she gave birth to twins. Initially, Perry had rushed to see to Mrs Nicholson in an emergency situation, as she had started to give birth and neither Jones nor the other doctors of the practice had been available at the time. However, Jones, being busy the following days as well, allowed his assistant to visit her two more times after the birth, which appeared to have been uncomplicated, and also to take care of the official notification of birth form, in which Perry inserted Jones's name as the doctor attending. When Jones eventually followed a call to personally visit Mrs Nicholson four days after the birth, she had developed puerperal fever. Though transferred immediately to a local workhouse infirmary, where retained pieces of placenta were removed, she died there a few days later. On learning about the case, Sheffield's Medical Officer of Health contacted the coroner, who – following a personal request of the widower, Mr Nicholson – arranged for an exhumation of the already buried body. The post-mortem examination indicated that Mrs Nicholson had died from

[60] General Council, 'Medical Disciplinary Cases', p. 340.

'purely natural causes', which 'would include puerperal septicaemia [blood poisoning]',[61] and that there were no injuries caused by the delivery. Still, the Medical Officer of Health ensured that the case went, via the British Medical Association as complainant, to the GMC.[62] After hearing Jones and witnesses, and considering depositions from individuals involved in the case, the GMC found Jones guilty of infamous conduct in a professional respect and erased his name from the Register.[63] His name was restored 30 months later.[64]

The Day–Davenport case and the Jones–Perry case thus illustrate how the issue of employing unqualified assistants was bound up with suspicions of incompetent practice – even though in the former case family members of the deceased declared during the inquest that they had always been satisfied with 'Dr Davenport', and in the latter case, Jones provided evidence that members of Mrs Nicholson's family had continued to see him as their doctor after her death.[65] Employing and covering unqualified assistants was seen as a professional offence not only because it precluded employment opportunities for qualified junior practition-

[61] Ibid., p. 342.
[62] Ibid., pp. 340-347.
[63] Ibid., p. 347; *Minutes*, vol. 47, 1910, pp. 46-48.
[64] Smith, *Medical Discipline*, p. 253.
[65] *Minutes*, vol. 23, 1886, p. 117; General Council, 'Medical Disciplinary Cases', p. 344.

ers, but also because it could involve serious danger for patients. By the mid-1920s the position of the GMC on the issue was unmistakably clear. As barristers William Sanderson and E. B. A. Rayner warned in their textbook on legal aspects of medical practice:

> The General Medical Council regards the employment of an unqualified person as an assistant, as fraudulent and dangerous to the public interest, and will take every step in its power to prevent or punish practitioners who act in contravention of this rule. The Council is equally determined to suppress the practice of 'covering,' by which expression is meant countenancing or assisting an unqualified or unregistered person to attend or treat patients.[66]

When, in 1906, GMC President Donald MacAlister commented on the influence of the Council on the development of medical professional ethics, he cited the issue of covering unqualified assistants as an example of effective intervention.[67] His other example was the issue of medical advertising, on which the GMC had expressed its disapproval in a resolution in 1899.[68] In late nineteenth-century Britain, medical advertising in newspapers and other forms of attracting patients, such as distribution of handbills or canvassing

---

[66] William Sanderson and E. B. A. Rayner, *An Introduction to the Law and Tradition of Medical Practice* (London, H. K. Lewis & Co., 1926), p. 29.

[67] MacAlister, 'General Medical Council', p. 819.

[68] Robert Saundby, *Medical Ethics: A Guide to Professional Conduct*, 2nd edn (London, Charles Griffin & Company, 1907), p. 128.

through health insurance societies, had become increasingly prevalent, linked to relative overcrowding of the profession and competition between practitioners. The medical establishment of the GMC, however, saw advertising as potentially 'infamous conduct'; not only was it perceived as unfair competition, but coming from the world of trade, standing in the tradition of quackery, and often being linked with unorthodox treatments, it was regarded as profoundly ungentlemanly and as endangering the profession's reputation.[69]

The issue had been long-standing. Since the late 1850s the medical journal the *Lancet* had regularly published complaints of medical practitioners about colleagues' 'unprofessional' circulars or frequently repeated newspaper advertisements for their services or book publications, and it had commented that such tradesman-like conduct was lowering the profession's standing in the eyes of the public.[70] In 1871 a *Lancet* editorial complained that the medical corporations,

---

[69] Morrice, '"Honour and Interests"', pp. 24-26; Jochen Binder, *Zwischen Standesrecht und Marktwirtschaft: Ärztliche Werbung zu Beginn des 20. Jahrhunderts im deutsch-englischen Vergleich* (Frankfurt/M., Peter Lang, 2000), pp. 75-83.

[70] 'Unprofessional Advertising', *The Lancet*, January 22, 1859, p. 101; 'Unprofessional Handbills', ibid., December 3, 1859, p. 578; 'Unprofessional Advertisements', ibid., November 9, 1861, p. 464; 'Professional Advertising', ibid., June 6, 1868, p. 731; 'Professional Advertising', ibid., February 6, 1869, p. 215; 'Professional Advertising', ibid., March 20, 1869, pp. 407-408; 'Unprofessional Advertising', ibid., May 29, 1869, p. 758; 'Unprofessional Advertising', ibid., June 5, 1869, p. 799; 'Unprofessional Advertising', ibid., June 19, 1869, p. 854.

in particular the Royal College of Surgeons of England and the Royal College of Physicians of London, did too little to discipline such behaviour of their fellows, members and licentiates, although they had appropriate powers and structures to do so.[71] By 1873 the Royal College of Surgeons had adopted a resolution condemning frequent advertising of medical works in the non-medical press, and the Royal College of Physicians had endorsed this resolution.[72] Also, the various forms of advertising were unmistakably censured in the medical deontological literature. As Jukes Styrap pointed out in his *A Code of Medical Ethics*:

> It is [...] derogatory to the profession to solicit practice by advertisement, circular, card, or placard; also, to offer, by public announcement, gratuitous advice to the poor, or to promise radical cures; to publish cases and operations in the daily press, or knowingly, to suffer such publications to be made; to advertise medical works in non-medical papers; to invite laymen to be present at operations; to boast of cures and remedies; to adduce testimonials of skill and success; or to do any like acts. Such are the ordinary practices of charlatans, and are incompatible with the honour and dignity of the pro-

[71] 'The Ethical Function of the Corporations', *The Lancet*, November 25, 1871, pp. 753-754.

[72] 'Professional Book Advertisements', *The Lancet,* December 21, 1872, p. 893; 'Medical Advertisements', ibid., May 17, 1873, pp. 711-712; 'Medical Advertising', ibid., June 28, 1873, p. 913.

> fession. [...] It is also extremely reprehensible for a practitioner to attest the efficacy of patent or secret medicines, or, in any way, to promote their use; only less culpable is the practice of written testimony in favour of articles of commerce, and tacitly or otherwise sanction its publication.[73]

However, the issue of medical advertising continued to cause concern. In 1879 the *Lancet* noted that scarcely a week passed 'without receiving communications from medical men who are annoyed by the paltry and unprofessional devices to which some of their neighbours resort to obtain public notice and "patronage".'[74] Unwilling to keep on publishing about individual cases of this kind, the journal resigned itself to the hope that the public would 'in the long run discover that the persons and the commodity that need so much advertising cannot be of great value or repute'.[75]

The *Medical Press and Circular*, however, took on the cause, pointing out in 1882 that a recent resolution by the Royal College of Physicians against advertising medical works in the lay press would remain entirely ineffective as long as the only consequence for perpetrators was loss of professional esteem. Only if the punishment consisted in loss of license, membership or fellowship of the College, a

---

[73] Styrap, *Code of Medical Ethics*, pp. 27-28.
[74] 'Medical Advertising', *The Lancet*, September 27, 1879, p. 485.
[75] Ibid.

measure that would then also be adopted by the other medical corporations, medical advertising would be stamped out.[76] Similarly, when the King and Queen's College of Physicians in Ireland passed later in the same year a resolution that described extensive advertising of medical works and giving 'laudatory certificates' of medicinal preparations and medical or surgical appliances as 'misleading to the public, derogatory to the dignity of the profession', and contrary to the College's traditions, the *Medical Press* criticised it as too vague and as 'impotent'.[77]

Yet, despite such worries, disciplinary action was taken in several cases. In 1887, for example, the Royal College of Surgeons in Ireland and the King and Queen's College of Physicians reported to the General Medical Council that they had withdrawn their diplomas from a practitioner, William Edward Robson, 'for having wilfully violated their regulations by publishing advertisements derogatory to the reputation, honour and dignity of the College'.[78] His name was erased from the GMC's Register but restored after 33 months.[79] A leading article in the *Medical Press* in the same year, pointed out that problematic self-advertisement occurred among professionally established practitioners as

---

[76] 'Advertisement as a Crime', *The Medical Press and Circular*, June 14, 1882, pp. 509-511.

[77] 'Medical Advertising', *The Medical Press and Circular*, November 8, 1882, p. 401.

[78] 'The Penalty of Advertising', *The Medical Press and Circular*, February 23, 1887, p. 183.

[79] Smith, *Medical Discipline*, p. 243.

well as 'the young and struggling', and was 'derogatory' anywhere, but 'doubly so when the daily bread is no longer at stake'.[80] In fact, in the following year a correspondent to the *Medical Press* accused even a member of the General Medical Council itself, the ophthalmic surgeon Robert Brudenell Carter, Fellow of the Royal College of Surgeons (FRCS), of publishing a 'glaring puff' for his dexterity and skill in the *Times* and the *Pall Mall Gazette*.[81]

Prominent in the GMC Minutes of the 1890s was the case of Dr Herbert Tibbits, a proponent and practitioner of the then controversial method of electrotherapy with weak currents.[82] The Royal College of Physicians of London had withdrawn his licentiateship and the Royal College of Physicians of Edinburgh his membership and fellowship, as he was deemed to have issued a 'laudatory certificate' on appliances of the Medical Battery Company. Tibbits protested against their decision in a letter to the GMC, pointing out

---

[80] 'Professional Advertising', *The Medical Press and Circular*, March 16, 1887, 246-247.

[81] M.R.C.S., '*The Times* as a Medium of Medical Advertisement', *The Medical Press and Circular*, September 5, 1888, p. 246. The issue of so-called indirect advertising by medical men who published on medical and health matters in the general press continued to exercise the GMC and the British Medical Association during the 1920s. See Andrew A. G. Morrice, '"The Medical Pundits": Doctors and Indirect Advertising in the Lay Press 1922-1927', *Medical History* 38 (1994), pp. 255-280.

[82] On 'medical electricians' in the Victorian period, including Tibbits, and electrotherapy's 'vexed status' between regular and irregular practice see Iwan Rhys Morus, 'Bodily Disciplines and Disciplined Bodies: Instruments, Skills and Victorian Electrotherapeutics', *Social History of Medicine* 19 (2006), pp. 241-259.

that he had merely made a pre-paid 'Report' to the Company after testing some of their appliances, but had not published the report himself.[83] Nevertheless, the GMC decided to hold an inquiry into his conduct and in December 1894 found him guilty of 'offences [...] infamous in a professional respect' and erased his name from the Register. His efforts in the following two years to have his name restored were unsuccessful.[84] In Tibbits' case it seems, the combination of product advertising ('laudatory certificate'), a link to a manufacturing company, and his support for an unorthodox or at least rather marginal form of treatment, went firmly against him.[85] It should be noted, though, that the 1858 Medical Act did not permit to erase a practitioner's name from the Register 'on the grounds of his having adopted any Theory of Medicine or Surgery'.[86]

Eventually, in 1905, a formal GMC Notice on advertising and canvassing described these methods as 'contrary to the public interest and discreditable to the profession of medicine' and warned that any practitioner resorting to such practices rendered himself liable to the charge of 'infamous

---

[83] *Minutes*, vol. 31, 1894, pp. 70-74.

[84] *Minutes*, vol. 31, 1894, pp. 74, 153-154,156-157; vol. 33, 1896, pp. 232-237.

[85] Advertising, in particular self-advertisement, had also provided the grounds for the erasure from the Register of naturopath and anti-vaccinationist doctor Thomas Richard Allinson in 1892; see *Minutes*, vol. 26, 1889, pp. 211-218; vol. 29, 1892, pp. 75, 79-81, 154. For a full discussion of Allinson's case, see P. S. Brown, 'Medically Qualified Naturopaths and the General Medical Council', *Medical History* 35 (1991), pp. 50-77.

[86] Cited ibid., p. 54.

conduct in a professional respect' and might have his name erased from the Register if found guilty.[87] As GMC member and Vice President of the British Medical Association, Robert Saundby, explained in his booklet *Medical Ethics: A Guide to Professional Conduct* in 1907:

> No medical practitioner should seek publicity by advertisement except in certain recognized ways, as to do so is to attempt to get practice by other than the legitimate means of proficiency in his profession and skill or success in dealing with his patients. The only advertisement to the public now permissible is the door-plate [...].[88]

Between 1900 and 1914 advertising and canvassing belonged to the most common disciplinary offences. From a total of 206 disciplinary cases dealt with by the GMC during this period, 23 concerned advertising and 18 canvassing.[89] Again, as in the matter of covering unqualified assistants (which still concerned 26 cases in the same period), the Council's disciplinary stance derived not only from professional self-interest (i.e. the intention to mitigate competition) but also from a claim to protect the public against unscrupulous practice. As Saundby maintained, the lay public was unable to judge, for example, the value of advertised patent medicines, and he warned:

---

[87] *Minutes,* vol. 42, 1905, pp. 249-250; Saundby, *Medical Ethics*, p. 129. See also MacAlister, 'General Medical Council', p. 819.

[88] Saundby, *Medical Ethics*, p. 3.

[89] Smith, *Medical Discipline*, pp. 248-255.

If medical practitioners advertised [...] [t]here would be in consequence a general lowering of the standard of the profession, its ranks would be crowded with sharp business men, and the true scientific worker would be elbowed out and starved, until the public found out, as it might do after long years, that a bold liar is not a trustworthy medical adviser [...].[90]

Conclusions

From the variety of cases discussed in this chapter it is clear that in the nineteenth and early twentieth centuries the GMC was concerned about two broad matters: the moral conduct of practitioners and the safeguarding of qualified practice. Disciplinary actions in these areas were taken in the interest of patients and the public, based on the legal remit that was given to the Council in the Medical Act of 1858. Some of the measures taken, in particular against unqualified practice and against medical advertising, also favoured interests of qualified, orthodox and established practitioners, as one would expect from a body that was composed of this type of practitioner. A shortcoming of the GMC was that it had no direct control over medical performance, only indirectly through the monitoring of educational standards and practitioners' qualifications. To its credit, the GMC at-

90 Saundby, *Medical Ethics*, pp. 5-6.

tempted through its disciplinary role to ensure that the public could receive treatment from trustworthy and competent medical practitioners. However, this system of professional self-regulation and discipline had serious weaknesses, as became obvious in the second half of the twentieth century, especially in the 1990s with the Bristol paediatric heart surgery scandal and with the case of medical serial killer Harold Shipman.[91] Since then, the GMC, for a time fearing for its continued existence, has made considerable efforts to ensure safe medical practice for the public, for example by the creation of a Medical Practitioners Tribunal Service, which is still part of the GMC but answerable to Parliament, and by introducing a revalidation of practitioners scheme.[92] The long-term effects of these changes, which were implemented from 2012, remain to be seen. However, from a historical perspective, it would be unfair to doubt the GMC's foundational intention to serve the interests of patients and the public at large as well as to protect the interests of qualified medical practitioners. The practice of medical ethics in

[91] Stacey, *Regulating British Medicine*; M. Stacey, 'The General Medical Council and Professional Self-Regulation', in David Gladstone (ed.), *Regulating Doctors* (London, Institute for the Study of Civil Society, 2000), pp. 28-39; Donald Irvine, *The Doctors' Tale: Professionalism and Public Trust* (Abingdon, Radcliffe Medical Press, 2003), pp. 121-135, 161-172.

[92] Irvine, *Doctors' Tale*, pp. 139-159, 183-184; Roz Sullivan, 'All Changed: Changed Utterly – The Disciplinary Process of the GMC, 1858-2012', *The Scottish Society of the History of Medicine, Report of Proceedings*, Session 2012-2013 and 2013-2014 [publ. 2016], pp. 4-8.

the nineteenth century, as reflected in the disciplinary activities of the GMC, was more patient-oriented than has been generally assumed in the age of bioethics. In that sense, the history of medicine suggests that modern bioethics was less of an innovation than has been claimed.

Chapter 2

Doctor–Patient Communication and the Questions of Consent and Truth

Introduction

The question to what extent nineteenth-century doctors informed their patients and sought their explicit consent before treatment remains notoriously difficult to answer. In the early 1980s, the heyday of Anglo-American debates on informed consent, the historical interpretations of physician and law professor Jay Katz and historian Martin Pernick clashed. While Katz described a 'silent world' in which paternalistic physicians expected patients to trust them without questions, Pernick aimed to show that in America consent-seeking was part of an 'indigenous medical tradition' already in the nineteenth century.[93] More recent studies by Kathleen Powderly on the USA, Karen Nolte on Germany,

[93] Jay Katz, *The Silent World of Doctor and Patient* (New York, The Free Press, 1986); Martin Pernick, 'The Patient's Role in Medical Decisionmaking: A Social History of Informed Consent in Medical Therapy', in: President's Commission for the Study of Ethical Problems in Medicine and Biomedical and Behavioral Research, *Making Health Care Decisions*, vol. 3 (1982), pp. 1-35.

and Sally Wilde on Britain, Australia, and New Zealand have pointed to various forms of 'negotiation' between nineteenth-century doctors and their patients, especially if a risky treatment or mutilating operation was proposed.[94]

This chapter focuses on an English legal case from the 1890s, *Beatty v. Cullingworth,* which demonstrates that even if a patient was – at least to some extent – informed and the proposed treatment discussed, consent could be a contested issue. In 1896, Alice Beatty, a professional nurse, accused the senior obstetric physician of St. Thomas's Hospital London, Charles Cullingworth, of having removed her ovaries without her consent. The various dimensions of this case – professional ethics, law, gender, and the history of gynaecological surgery – add to its complexity. So, apart from the details of this case, I will highlight some specific contexts. However, I also want to argue that the key to its understanding and to the historical problem of consent more generally lies in the nineteenth-century medical tradition of truth-telling, a topic which was usually treated separately in the historical medical ethics literature.

---

[94] Kathleen E. Powderly, 'Patient Consent and Negotiation in the Brooklyn Gynecological Practice of Alexander J. C. Skene: 1863-1900', *Journal of Medicine and Philosophy* 25 (2000), pp. 12-27; Karen Nolte, 'Zeitalter des ärztlichen Paternalismus? – Überlegungen zu Aufklärung und Einwilligung von Patienten im 19. Jahrhundert', *Medizin, Gesellschaft und Geschichte* 25 (2007), pp. 59-89; Sally Wilde, 'Truth, Trust, and Confidence in Surgery, 1890-1910': Patient Autonomy, Communication, and Consent', *Bulletin of the History of Medicine* 83 (2009), pp. 302-330.

The Case of *Beatty v. Cullingworth*

In August 1892, Miss Beatty consulted Dr Cullingworth on advice of her sister, a nurse at St. Thomas's Home, because of a swelling in the pelvis, which he diagnosed as an inflamed cyst of the right ovary. In line with then current practice, he advised that it was necessary to operate and remove the tumour. Whether the ovary of the other side was healthy he could not be sure until he could view it during the operation. Miss Beatty did not want to take the risk of losing both ovaries, thus becoming infertile, as she was engaged to be married, and so she initially refused the proposed operation. Subsequently, however, she appeared to have agreed, via the then head of St. Thomas's Home, Mr Bidwell, to be operated on. In a further consultation on the next day, Cullingworth said that he could not promise not to remove the second ovary if this turned out to be necessary. Nevertheless, the operation went ahead the following morning. Beforehand, when brought into the operation room, Miss Beatty repeated that she did not wish to lose both her ovaries. If both were found to be diseased, she wanted neither of them removed. Cullingworth assured her that he knew her wishes; that he would not remove more than what was necessary; and that she really had to leave the matter in his hands. Beatty got onto the operating table and took the anaesthetic. During the operation Cullingworth removed the right ovary with a large cyst the size of two fists. The left ovary was found to be the size of a hen's egg and to also have a cyst. He first punctured the cyst to collapse it, then, on finding a blood clot and beginning suppuration in it, tried to dissect it out of the ovary; but as only a shell of ovarian tissue would remain, he entirely removed the left ovary as well.[95]

Having recuperated from the operation and having learnt about its extent, Beatty took legal action against Cullingworth for damages because of negligence, charging him with wrongfully removing her ovaries, also with wrongfully detaining them, exhibiting them and lecturing on them. She later dropped this action, however, on her counsel's advice. Cullingworth did not charge fees for the operation. In July 1893, Beatty went to Cullingworth's house, told him that the lawsuit had been dropped and asked him to arrange a job for her as a nurse because she had found no employment since her operation almost a year ago. When she refused his repeated requests to leave his house, Cullingworth allegedly first threatened to call a psychiatrist to have her committed to a lunatic asylum, but then returned with a police constable who, together with Cullingworth, forcefully removed her from the house and took her to a police station where Cullingworth charged her with entering his house and persistently annoying him. The magistrate

95 'Beatty v. Cullingworth', *British Medical Journal*, November 21, 1896, pp. 1525-1526; 'Beatty versus Cullingworth', *The Lancet*, November 21, 1896, pp. 1473-1474.

hearing the case dismissed the charges. Miss Beatty, however, sued Cullingworth for assault and a malicious prosecution. The outcome of this trial was that Miss Beatty was awarded only notional damages worth one farthing, but Cullingworth, besides paying 20 shillings into Court for her compensation, had to bear the considerable legal expenses for his defence.[96]

In 1896, finally, Beatty entered a fresh action against Cullingworth for having removed her ovaries without her consent and also for having prevented her from getting employment at several specified institutions. While the latter charge was subsequently withdrawn, the case was heard in court. About the question whether the removal of the left ovary had been justified, the most eminent gynaecological surgeons of that time, Robert Lawson Tait (1845–1899) and Sir Thomas Spencer Wells (1818–1897), were heard as expert witnesses for opposite sides. On the crucial question of whether Cullingworth had operated with *tacit* consent, however, the jury came to the conclusion that he had, thus exonerating him.[97]

---

[96] 'Beatty v. Cullingworth', *The Times*, April 11, 1894, p. 3.

[97] 'Beatty v. Cullingworth', *British Medical Journal*, November 21, 1896, pp. 1525-1526; 'Beatty versus Cullingworth', *The Lancet*, November 21, 1896, pp. 1473-1474.

Contexts of the Case

Apart from the gendered nature of gynaecological surgery itself, the gender issue, in an era of developing feminism, is apparent in Beatty's repeated attempts to obtain compensation for what she regarded as an injury, but what her male doctor saw as a life-saving operation. The high-handed, as well as paternalistic, behaviour of Cullingworth corresponded to contemporary gender stereotypes and to the self-confidence of surgeons in a period when anaesthetics (since the mid-1840s), antisepsis (from the late 1860s), and greater attention to cleanliness, had much increased the scope and success of operations. Ovariotomy (i.e. the excising of ovaries), an operation introduced in 1809, came to stand for progress in nineteenth-century surgery. Yet, it had an ambiguous status in the 1890s. Following considerable intra-professional controversy due to the operation's high risk of death in the early and middle decades of the nineteenth century, it had become, by the 1890s, an established treatment for ovarian tumours or cysts (as in Miss Beatty's case), which were seen as otherwise incurable, eventually leading to death. However, the operation had been more widely carried out in the late 1870s and 1880s to eliminate ovarian function as a treatment for menstrual pains, hysterical fits and epilepsy, and various other nervous or mental disorders which were thought to be connected with the female reproductive organs. The removal of seemingly normal ovaries for those conditions, or 'Battey's operation', named after the American surgeon Robert Battey who had introduced this treatment approach in 1872, had become fashionable in the United States and Britain, but began to lose its popularity at the end of the nineteenth century. There were contemporary concerns, even among ovariotomists themselves, that some surgeons might be too rash in extirpating ovaries, in this way 'unsexing' women, i.e. not only making them sterile but also depriving them of female sexual feeling.[98] By 1910, the New York physician Norman Batesby forcefully denounced the 'gynaecological perverts', as he called them, who seemed to enjoy performing ovariotomies whenever they had an opportunity for it.[99]

To be sure, Cullingworth did not carry out ovariotomy on Miss Beatty for those controversial reasons, but there were overtones of this connection when he had her forcefully removed from his house as an apparently insane

---

[98] Ornella Moscucci, *The Science of Woman: Gynaecology and Gender in England, 1800-1929* (Cambridge, New York and Melbourne: Cambridge University Press, 1993), pp. 134-164; Ann Dally, *Women under the Knife: A History of Surgery* (Edison, NJ: Castle Books, 2006), pp. 147-156; eadem, *Fantasy Surgery, 1880-1930: with special reference to Sir William Arbuthnot Lane* (Amsterdam and Atlanta, Rodopi, 1996), pp. 20-27; Sally Frampton, 'Defining Difference: Competing Forms of Ovarian Surgery in the Nineteenth Century', in Thomas Schlich and Christopher Crenner (eds), *Technological Change in Modern Surgery: Historical Perspectives on Innovation* (Rochester, NY, University of Rochester Press, 2017), pp. 51-70.

[99] Norman Batesby, *Medical Chaos and Crime* (London and New York, Mitchell Kennerley, 1910), pp. 230-252.

woman. Closer to Cullingworth's case, the need for ovariotomy operations had been contested also regarding some physical (not mental) conditions. In 1886, Francis Imlach, an obstetrician at Liverpool's Hospital for Women, had been sued for damages by one of his patients, Mrs Mary Casey (and her husband John, a labourer and former sailor), for having removed her ovaries and Fallopian tubes without medical necessity and without her consent. Imlach was found not guilty, as the head nurse, Sarah White, stated that Mrs Casey had been informed by Imlach about the nature of the planned operation and that she, White, herself had told her about it on the morning of the operation. Yet the trial revealed differences of opinion among the medical experts regarding the need for operative treatment of her condition, which had been diagnosed by Imlach as haematosalpinx and haematocele, i.e. an accumulation of blood in and around the tubes. Although the majority of the medical expert witnesses supported Imlach's decision to operate, the case led to renewed medical and public debate about the purposes of radical ovarian surgery more generally.[100] A year later, Imlach's colleague at the Liverpool Hospital for Women, the surgeon J. E. Burton (who had been listed as a witness for the plaintiff but then had not appeared for the trial) addressed the International Medical Congress in Washington about the indications for removing the ovaries,

[100] 'The Action against Dr. Imlach, of Liverpool', *British Medical Journal*, August 21, 1886, pp. 394-395; Moscucci, *Science of Woman*, pp.160-164.

or, as he called it 'castration of women' or 'spaying'. In his view such a serious operation, amounting to 'mutilation' and 'degradation' of women, violated the Hippocratic rule to do no harm, unless it was performed in justified cases (which he detailed) after conservative medical treatments had failed; following consultation with colleagues; and after 'full explanation of the nature of the proposed operation and its results to the patient herself and her nearest friend (husband, mother or father).' For haematocele and haematosalpinx the removal of the ovaries and tubes was in his opinion not justifiable under any conditions.[101]

More generally, the image of gynaecological surgery in Britain, as a field, may still have suffered not only from the controversies over the risks and consequences of ovariotomy but also from the scandal around London surgeon Isaac Baker Brown in the late 1860s. He had performed numerous clitoridectomy operations on women with epilepsy and mental problems, on the assumption that these disorders were caused by female masturbation (for which removal of the clitoris was seen by him as the obvious cure). Often, it seems, Brown had carried out 'his' operation without beforehand telling the women, or their husbands, what

---

[101] J. E. Burton, 'When Shall We Operate in Ovarian and Tubal Inflammations?', *The Medical Press and Circular* 95 (1887), pp. 291-292.

exactly he was going to do. Eventually, he had been expelled for misconduct from his professional association, the Obstetrical Society of London.[102]

Legally, operations without consent could in principle be regarded as assault and battery. This aspect was probably less discussed in Britain than on the European continent, where a German Supreme Court decision in 1894, just two years before Cullingworth's acquittal, had confirmed this legal view in the case of a Hamburg surgeon who had operated on a child against the explicit wishes of her father.[103]

Two English precedents on surgical procedures without consent, *Slater v. Baker and Stapleton* (1767) and *Absolon v. Statham* (1866), were dealt with by the courts as malpractice cases rather than as cases of assault.[104] In the first case, Baker, a surgeon at St. Bartholomew's Hospital in London, was mulcted in damages for £500, as he had – assisted by

---

[102] Dally, *Women under the Knife*, pp. 160-184; Phil Fennel, *Treatment without Consent: Law, psychiatry and the treatment of mentally disordered people since 1845* (London and New York, Routledge, 1996), pp. 66-72; Moscucci, *Science of Woman*, p. 105; Andrew Scull, *Hysteria: The Biography* (Oxford and New York, Oxford University Press, 2009), pp. 76-83.

[103] See Andreas-Holger Maehle, *Doctors, Honour and the Law: Medical Ethics in Imperial Germany* (Basingstoke, Palgrave Macmillan, 2009), pp. 74-76.

[104] John J. Elwell, *A Medico-Legal Treatise on Malpractice and Medical Evidence, Comprising the Elements of Medical Jurisprudence* (New York, John S. Voorhies, 1860), pp. 112-115; Alexander Young, 'The Law of Malpractice', *Boston Medical and Surgical Journal*, new series, 5 (1870), pp. 425-443; 'Medical Trials. Absolon v. Statham', *The Lancet*, November 17, 1866, pp. 561-564; Pernick, 'The Patient's Role', pp. 15, 24; Ruth R. Faden and Tom L. Beauchamp in collaboration with Nancy M. P. King, *A History and Theory of Informed Consent* (New York and Oxford, Oxford University Press, 1986), pp. 116-117.

the apothecary, Stapleton – re-fractured Mr Slater's healing broken leg against his explicit wishes, in order to treat the leg fracture in a novel extension apparatus. The judge, Chief Justice Wilmot, characterised Baker's way of proceeding in this case as rash, ignorant, and unskilful, i.e. as negligent.[105] In the second case, Mrs Absolon, a dressmaker, accused a London surgeon, Mr Statham, of assault as he had administered chloroform to her and then extracted six of her teeth, although she had previously objected to both the tooth extraction and the anaesthetic (having had a bad reaction to chloroform at an earlier occasion). In the trial, however, the focus was less on the question of consent than on Mrs Absolon's condition, which was described by an expert witness as neuralgic pains, and the appropriateness of giving chloroform despite her pre-history, and of extracting six teeth in one session. The jury was unable to agree a verdict and was discharged.[106]

Although patient complaints about medical practitioners were common throughout the nineteenth century, especially in the context of medical care under the Poor Law, cases of litigation such as the two above were rare, as high

---

[105] Young, 'Law of Malpractice', pp. 432-433.
[106] 'Absolon v. Statham', pp. 561-564.

legal costs tended to be an obstacle for patients and doctors alike.[107]

Moreover, surgical interventions without consent in life-threatening emergencies were regarded as justified. This was demonstrated by the acquittal of a medical officer at the Shadwell Children's Hospital, London, in 1890. He had performed a tracheotomy on a 13-month-old child suffering from an obstruction of the windpipe, although the child's mother had refused her consent to the operation. The child having died shortly after the intervention, a coroner's inquest was held which fully vindicated the doctor's operation without parental consent as the only chance he then had to save the child's life. As the coroner even put it, if the doctor had *not* performed the operation because he lacked the parents' consent, some juries might have found him guilty of manslaughter.[108]

In the British context, the seeking of consent was more seen as a matter of professional prudence and custom than a strict legal requirement, as the comments of the *British Medical Journal* and the *Lancet* on the Cullingworth case indicated. As the *BMJ* stated:

---

[107] See Kim Price, 'The shape of the iceberg: Doctors and neglect under the New Poor Law, c. 1871-1900', in: Jonathan Reinarz and Rebecca Wynter (eds), *Complaints, Controversies and Grievances in Medicine: Historical and social science perspectives* (London and New York, Routledge, 2015), pp. 129-146; Steven King, 'The role of complaint in establishing the rights of the patient and the duties of the doctor', ibid., pp. 149-166.

[108] 'The Right to Perform Operations in Hospitals', *British Medical Journal*, March 1, 1890, pp. 496-497.

> Had Dr Cullingworth got a written consent to the performance of such an operation as he thought right, or even a verbal consent given in unequivocal terms before witnesses, all the subsequent trouble would have been avoided. The moral is: Before doing an operation surgeons should be careful to explain what they propose to do, and get unequivocal consent from the patient, or, if the patient is not in a condition to give consent, from the patient's nearest friends. Such consent should be either in writing or distinctly expressed before witnesses.[109]

The *Lancet*'s comment was similar but steeped in medical paternalism:

> It is no doubt always advisable, especially where operations are in question, to endeavour to put clearly before the patient what the risk of the operation is, and what effects, beneficial or otherwise, may be expected to result from it. But it is a matter of common knowledge how often seemingly plain explanations of this kind are more or less completely misunderstood. Consent or refusal should be the only terms recognised in questions of operation. The patient cannot expect to do more than grasp the outline of what is in contemplation, and must be content to leave it to the discretion and judgement of the operator to fill in the details as may seem to him best.[110]

[109] 'Beatty v. Cullingworth', *British Medical Journal*, November 21, 1896, p. 1525.

[110] 'Beatty versus Cullingworth', *The Lancet*, November 21, 1896, p. 1474.

However, was the seeking of consent, as this comment suggests, merely hampered by insufficient lay understandings of surgical or medical procedures? Was it simply a matter of 'doctor knows best', as one might assume? There was much in Cullingworth's conduct that supports this interpretation, though his case was more complicated as his patient, Miss Beatty, was also a health professional, albeit not a doctor, and had clearly expressed her wishes before she mounted the operating table.

For the American context, the opinion of Justice Benjamin Cardozo in the case of *Schloendorff v. Society of New York Hospitals* (1914) has often been cited as heralding patient consent as a feature of a person's right to self-determination. Mrs Schloendorff had consented to an abdominal examination under anaesthesia, but had explicitly asked not to have an operation. Nevertheless, her surgeon operatively removed a fibroid tumour. As Justice Cardozo stated:

> Every human being of adult years and sound mind has a right to determine what shall be done with his own body; and a surgeon who performs an operation without his patient's consent commits an assault, for which he is liable in damages.[111]

---

[111] Cited in Faden and Beauchamp, *History and Theory of Informed Consent*, p. 123.

With regard to the Cullingworth case, however, a key to understanding the consent problem lies, I would like to suggest, in another aspect of nineteenth-century doctor–patient dialogues, namely truth-telling.

Truth at the Sickbed

In contrast to consent, truth-telling, particularly in terminally ill patients, was a regular topic in the historical medical ethics literature. Edinburgh professor of medicine John Gregory, for example, included this subject in his influential *Lectures on the Duties and Qualifications of a Physician*, published in 1772. Gregory raised the question of truth-telling for the situation that a patient's illness was so serious that his or her life was in danger. In these circumstances, he believed, a deviation from the truth was 'both justifiable and necessary', as an extremely ill patient might still recover if not informed about the danger. However, the patient's relatives should be told about the real situation, particularly if the patient still needed to settle financial affairs. It also gave the relatives the opportunity to call for further assistance.[112] The idea was that patients should not be deprived of hope by learning the full truth about their condition. This advice to doctors conflicted to some extent with Gregory's general expectation that they should feel bound to truthfulness or

---

112 John Gregory, *Lectures on the Duties and Qualifications of a Physician* (London, W. Strahan and T. Cadell, 1772), pp. 34-35.

'candour', in the sense of being ready to acknowledge errors and to rectify mistakes in treatment.[113] The tension between being truthful as a medical gentleman and a willingness to bend the truth to avoid harmful anxiety of the patient was sharply perceived in the mid-1790s by a non-medical writer on professional ethics, the Reverend Thomas Gisborne:

> The Physician may not be bound, unless expressly called upon, invariably to divulge at any specific time his opinion concerning the uncertainty or danger of the case: but he is invariably bound never to represent the uncertainty or danger as less than he actually believes it to be; and whenever he conveys, directly or indirectly, to the patient or to his family, any impression to that effect, though he may be misled by mistaken tenderness, he is guilty of positive falsehood. He is at liberty to say little; but let that little be true. St. Paul's direction, *not to do evil that good may come,* is clear, positive, and universal.[114]

In Gisborne's opinion, in contrast to Gregory's, the truth should not be sacrificed out of concern for the patient's feelings. In practical terms, however, his advice was quite similar to that given by Gregory, whom he acknowledged as an influence. If the situation of the patient was critical, some of the patient's near relations should be informed about this,

---

[113] Ibid., pp. 28-29.

[114] Thomas Gisborne, *An Enquiry into the Duties of Men in the Higher and Middle Classes of Society in Great Britain, Resulting from their Respective Stations, Professions, and Employments*, 3rd edition (London, B. and J. White, 1795), vol. 2, p. 149.

and the patient or his friends might have to be advised about 'the propriety of adjusting all unfinished temporal concerns' (i.e. the patient should be induced to make his last will). The physician might also discreetly turn the patient's thoughts towards religion, preparing in this way the entry of the clergyman.[115]

Manchester physician Thomas Percival, who had circulated in 1794 a manuscript version of his later book *Medical Ethics* (1803) to friends and colleagues, was another acknowledged influence on Gisborne.[116] More importantly, Percival's book served as the blueprint for the *Code of Ethics* of the American Medical Association, adopted in 1847, and became influential on nineteenth-century British writers about medical ethics.[117] Regarding truth-telling, he advised that in life-threatening illnesses the patient's friends should be informed about the danger, but the patient only 'if absolutely necessary'. In this case the bad news should be communicated by a suitable person other than the doctor, so that, as Percival claimed, the doctor could maintain his role

---

[115] Ibid., pp. 121, 150-151.

[116] Ibid., p. 121. On the writing of Percival's book and its specific contexts in Manchester, see John V. Pickstone, 'Thomas Percival and the Production of Medical Ethics', in: Robert Baker, Dorothy Porter and Roy Porter (eds), *The Codification of Medical Morality*, vol. 1: *Medical Ethics and Etiquette in the Eighteenth Century* (Dordrecht, Kluwer Academic Publishers, 1993, pp. 161-178.

[117] Robert Baker, 'Deciphering Percival's Code', ibid., pp. 179-211.

as 'the minister of hope and comfort to the sick', lift the patient's depressed mood and 'smooth the bed of death'.[118] Percival's advice to medical practitioners was thus to *evade* disclosing a dire prognosis in such situations, rather than bending the truth. This was in line with Gisborne's admonition not to lie at the sickbed, a point about which Gisborne had explicitly written to Percival,[119] but the latter also adopted Gregory's advice to involve the patient's relatives in cases of terminal illness. Percival had been sufficiently exercised by the problem of truth-telling to study the opinions of various authoritative writers on the subject, finding contradictory advice, e.g. Glasgow philosopher Frances Hutcheson asserting that 'No man censures a physician for deceiving a patient too much dejected, by expressing good hopes of him', while the writer Samuel Johnson denied the right to lie to a patient out of fear of alarming him, insisting that 'You have no business with consequences…you are to tell the truth'.[120] In his own analysis of the issue, Percival distinguished moral truth delivered to another party (i.e. the patient) and moral truth towards oneself (i.e. the physician). In extreme circumstances, such as serious illness of a

---

[118] Thomas Percival, 'Medical Ethics; or, a Code of Institutes and Precepts, Adapted to the Professional Conduct of Physicians and Surgeons' (1803), in: Chauncey D. Leake (ed.), *Percival's Medical Ethics* (Huntington, NY, Robert E. Krieger Publishing Company, 1975), pp. 61-205, on p. 91.

[119] Cited ibid., pp. 186-187.

[120] Cited ibid., pp. 191, 193.

father of a numerous family or of a person of great importance to the community, the physician should sacrifice his personal moral sense of veracity in the interest of his social duty and therefore not reveal the truth which might kill the patient.[121]

Percival also briefly discussed how to behave towards a patient undergoing an operation (in the pre-anaesthetic era):

> A decorous silence ought to be observed. It may be humane and salutary, however, for one of the attending physicians or surgeons to speak occasionally to the patient; to comfort him under his sufferings, and to give him assurance, if consistent with truth, that the operation goes on well, and promises a speedy and successful termination.[122]

In other words, for Percival, keeping the patient informed in critical situations was only advisable if some beneficial effect could be expected from it, otherwise the medical practitioner should remain silent. Moreover, when physicians and surgeons jointly examined a patient, for example in hospital in advance of an operation, 'the particular circumstances of danger or difficulty should be carefully concealed from him, and every just precaution used to guard him from anxiety and alarm.'[123]

---

[121] Ibid., pp. 194-195.
[122] Ibid., p. 82.
[123] Ibid., pp. 81-82.

In 1836, Michael Ryan, an Irish-born lecturer in medicine and midwifery in London, continued this line of advice in his *Manual of Medical Jurisprudence and State Medicine*. Claiming that 'a tone, a word, a look will destroy life in delicate and dangerous cases', he acknowledged that 'official' mendacity, i.e. in the role of physician, was less pernicious than 'malicious' mendacity, but pointed to the general injunction not to do evil, that good may follow. Following Christian morality, Ryan admonished never to promise recovery without premising that it depended on 'Divine will' as well as on adherence to the medical precepts, and he advised to express any prognosis with greatest caution.[124] In addition, he reprinted the passages on truth-telling in seriously ill patients from Gregory and Percival.[125]

Percival's advice on truth-telling was adopted, like much else from his *Medical Ethics*, by the American Medical Association for their *Code of Ethics* of 1847. Similarly as Ryan's manual, the AMA code in addition emphasized the risk that even the words and manner of a physician betraying a gloomy prognosis might shorten the life of a seriously ill patient. Therefore, such depressing conduct had to be

[124] Michael Ryan, 'A Manual of Medical Jurisprudence and State Medicine' (1836), in: Howard Brody, Zahra Meghani and Kimberly Greenwald (eds), *Michael Ryan's Writings on Medical Ethics* (Dordrecht, Springer, 2010), pp. 79-222, on pp. 134-135.

[125] Ibid., pp. 148, 168.

carefully avoided.[126] The AMA code, in turn, served with minor alterations as the source for the section on truth-telling in the *Code of Medical Ethics* (1878) by the Shrewsbury physician Jukes Styrap. This English code went through three further editions until 1895, and was described in 1896 by the *British Medical Journal* as 'the usually accepted authority on ethics of the BMA'.[127] As Styrap advised on the issue of truth-telling:

> A practitioner should not be prone to make gloomy prognostications, inasmuch as, they not only exert a depressive influence on the invalid, but savour strongly of empiricism by unduly magnifying the importance of his services in the treatment or cure of the disease; at the same time, he should not fail to give to the friends of the patient timely notice of actual danger, and even to the patient himself, if absolutely necessary, or when specially desired by the relatives. The communication, however, when personally made by the doctor, is generally so alarming to the patient that, whenever it can, it had better be delegated to some discreet relative, or other sympathising friend; for the medical attendant should be the minister of hope and comfort to the sick – that, by

---

[126] Isaac Hayes, 'Code of Ethics', in: Robert Baker (ed.), *The Codification of Medical Morality*, vol. 2: *Anglo-American Medical Ethics and Medical Jurisprudence in the Nineteenth Century* (Dordrecht, Kluwer Academic Publishers, 1995), pp. 75-87, on p. 76.

[127] Cited in Peter Bartrip, 'An Introduction to Jukes Styrap's *A Code of Medical Ethics* (1878)', in: Baker, *Codification of Medical Morality*, vol. 2, pp. 145-148, on p. 145.

> such cordials to the drooping spirit he may soothe the bed of death, revive expiring life, and counteract the depressing influence of those maladies which often disturb the tranquillity, even of the most resigned, in the trying moments of impending dissolution. Nor should it be forgotten that the ebbing life of a patient may be shortened not only by the acts, but also by the words and manner of the doctor; it is, therefore, his duty carefully to guard himself in this respect, and to avoid, as far as possible, everything which has a tendency to discourage the patient and depress his spirits.[128]

Some years before Styrap's statement, in 1869, the ethics of prognosis had been the topic of an editorial in the *Lancet*. While acknowledging that some doctors habitually tended to make gloomy prognoses and that some physicians believed that the patient should be told everything they knew and thought about the disease in hand, the editorial strongly advocated making a favourable prognosis whenever this was consistent with the facts. While a gloomy prognosis would do 'palpable harm' to the patient and hinder a cure, so the argument ran, putting the 'best construction' on symptoms might extend the patient's lifespan. Moreover, patients should not be troubled with information

[128] Jukes Styrap, *A Code of Medical Ethics* (London, J. & A. Churchill, 1878), p. 22.

which they were unable to fully understand and which might therefore mislead them.[129]

Through this line of tradition then, Percival's ethical stance of advocating only restricted disclosure to patients with a serious condition became standard in the medical profession at the time of the *Beatty v. Cullingworth* case, and it was propagated beyond that time into the twentieth century. As Robert Saundby stated in 1907, in the second edition of his guidebook *Medical Ethics*, a prognosis should in general be truthful but it was 'permissible to diminish the gravity of the case to a patient who is seriously ill, or to speak with perfect hopefulness in order to encourage a patient who may be suffering from a troublesome, though not a dangerous affection'. Only if patients insisted on knowing the truth, they should be informed. Otherwise, in serious cases, their family should be told the truth.[130]

Historian Pat Jalland has emphasized the common practice of Victorian physicians to use a family member of a dying patient to communicate, under their guidance, the truth about the terminal nature of the illness. Such indirect truth-telling was thought to be a doctor's moral duty in view of the perceived spiritual needs of the patient, although due to uncertainties in medical diagnosis physicians tended to be

[129] 'The Ethics of Prognosis', *The Lancet*, March, 13, 1869, pp. 366-367.
[130] Robert Saundby, *Medical Ethics: A Guide to Professional Conduct.* 2nd edn (London, Charles Griffin & Company, 1907), pp. 104-105, 117-118.

hesitant about making clear-cut prognostic statements.[131] While many terminally ill patients in the nineteenth century may eventually have learned about their prognosis in this indirect way, this practice rather confirms than undermines the notion of a medical tradition of restricted truth-telling in serious conditions in order to avoid harming the patient and to preserve hope in the doctor's treatments.

Conclusions

As these attitudes towards truth-telling during the long nineteenth century indicate, a culture of restricted information, in the presumed best interest of the patient, prevailed in the medical profession. While, by the late nineteenth century, doctors – or at least surgeons – became increasingly aware of the need to seek the patient's consent, in order to secure the patient's collaboration in the treatment effort and to avoid trouble, a long-ingrained habit of deliberately limiting what patients were told about the seriousness of their illness undermined the consent process. Patients' consent, if it was sought, was not fully informed, because doctors' fear of causing harm by telling the truth forbade them to enter a full and honest dialogue with their patients. Cullingworth had explained the medical condition to Miss Beatty, and the implications of potentially losing

131 Pat Jalland, *Death in the Victorian Family* (Oxford, Oxford University Press, 1996), pp. 108-118.

both her ovaries were obviously clear to her. But, it appears that he had not been outspoken about the prognosis of ovarian tumours which were known then to be almost always fatal, though many patients lived with them for years, suffering great discomfort as their tumour grew.[132] Escaping such a prognosis would, in Cullingworth's mind, have justified sacrificing Beatty's fertility. Although some kind of 'negotiation' preceded the operation, in the end 'silence' prevailed, and Cullingworth retracted to the paternalistic position that he would do what was necessary in the presumed best interest of his patient. This behaviour correlated to nineteenth-century medical practices of restricted truth-telling more generally. In other words, what a case such as *Beatty v. Cullingworth* revealed was the dominance of what bioethicists Ruth Faden and Tom Beauchamp have called the 'beneficence model' for consent-seeking and patient information.[133] Both practices were restricted by intentions to benefit the patient. Consent, under this model, served to improve the outcome of a treatment through patient cooperation; and information was only regarded as useful as long as it did not alarm and thereby harm the patient. The autonomy or self-determination of the patient in health-related decision-making was not yet a generally accepted concept –

[132] Frampton, 'Defining Difference', p. 53.
[133] Faden and Beauchamp, *History and Theory of Informed Consent,* pp. 59-60.

or, as Cullingworth so tellingly put it before operating on Miss Beatty: she really had to leave the matter in his hands.

Chapter 3

Writing about Medical Ethics: From John Gregory to Robert Saundby

Introduction

In considering the history of medical ethics there is a certain risk that present-day observers privilege those matters that resonate with current issues, at the cost of areas or approaches which were characteristic of their time and context. It is therefore useful to ask, and to explore in some detail, how historical authors conceptualised their writing on ethical matters in medicine and what *they* perceived as major ethical concerns. Starting with the published lectures of the eighteenth-century Scottish physician and Edinburgh professor John Gregory (1724-1773), I trace in this chapter British writings on medical ethics through the late eighteenth and nineteenth centuries, up to the 1907 guidance on professional conduct by Robert Saundby (1849–1918), a former president of the Council of the British Medical Association, which had been founded (as the Provincial Medical and Surgical Association) in 1832. In doing this I will show

how medical ethics developed from a matter of a doctor's personal integrity and gentlemanly behaviour to a broader concern over the professional reputation and responsibilities of medical practitioners in general.

Gregory: Characteristics of the Gentleman Doctor

A significant background to medical ethical writing in late eighteenth-century Britain was the hierarchy of practitioners, with the university-educated physicians at the top, followed by the apprenticeship- and hospital-trained surgeons and the apprenticeship-trained apothecaries. One concern addressed in the medical ethics literature of this time was, therefore, how physicians should interact with the two 'lower' groups of practitioners, in the interest of smooth professional relations as well as in the interest of patient care. When John Gregory, professor of the practice of medicine, gave c. 1770 his *Lectures on the Duties and Qualifications of a Physician* to his Edinburgh medical students, he addressed this hierarchy. While not denying the general educational superiority of physicians, he called for them to treat the other two groups with due respect, especially if they had obtained equivalent medical knowledge:

> Every department of it [i.e. the medical profession], is respectable, when exercised with capacity and integrity. I only contend for an evident truth, either that the different branches should be separately professed, or, if one

> person will profess all, he should be regularly educated to, and thoroughly master of all. [...] If a surgeon or apothecary has had the education, and acquired the knowledge of a physician, he is a physician to all intents and purposes, whether he has the degree or not, and ought to be respected and treated accordingly. In Great Britain, surgery is a liberal profession.[134]

Potential situations of professional conflict were consultations between practitioners over difficult cases. Here, according to Gregory, it had to be avoided to involve the patient in any quarrels. If a physician knew in advance that he would be unable to be open-minded about another medical practitioner's therapeutic suggestions, he should honourably decline the consultation.[135] However, the place of the other practitioner's university degree, or whether he had a degree at all, should play no role, nor the source of the proposed remedy. As Gregory emphasized:

> [...] I am not speaking here of the private police of a corporation, or the little arts of a craft. I am treating of the duties of a liberal profession, whose object is the life and health of the human species, a profession to be exercised by gentlemen of honour and ingenuous manners [...].[136]

---

[134] John Gregory, *Lectures on the Duties and Qualifications of a Physician. A New Edition, corrected and enlarged* (London, W. Strahan and T. Cadell, 1772), pp. 49-50. This publication was the authorised version of the lectures, approved by Gregory, after an unofficial version, based on student notes, had appeared in 1770. Cf. ibid., 'Advertisement'.

[135] Gregory, *Lectures*, pp. 36-37.

[136] Ibid., p. 39.

In other words, for Gregory the benefit to the patient was what counted in consultations, and professional rivalries had to be subordinated to this higher purpose. Medical practitioners should behave as gentlemen to each other, in the service of patient care.

Conduct in intra-professional relations was, however, only part of one of four areas of Gregory's broad approach to medical ethics. This approach comprised (1) the intellectual and temperamental qualities suited for being a physician, (2) the moral qualities expected from a practising physician, such as humanity, patience, attention, discretion, secrecy, and honour, in his dealings with his patients, (3) decorum and manners in his behaviour towards his patients and to other physicians, to surgeons, and to apothecaries, and (4) the education necessary to practise as a physician 'with success and reputation'.[137]

Concerning the first aspect, Gregory required a 'comprehensive' mind of a physician. In medicine, he believed, there was no established authority to which one could refer in doubtful cases, so every physician had to rely on 'his own judgement, which appeals for its rectitude to nature and experience alone'.[138] Gregory adopted here the Baconian ideal of observation and experiment as the (only) basis for the improvement of knowledge in science and medicine – a theme

[137] Ibid., pp. 11-12.
[138] Ibid., pp. 13-14.

on which he elaborated later on in his lectures. The physician needed 'a penetrating genius', 'a clear solid judgement', and often 'a quickness of apprehension' in order to perceive where the greatest probability of success lay in a case and to treat the patient accordingly.[139] Moreover, the physician had to be in command of his temper and passions, in order to be able to act quickly and resolutely in emergencies, even if he was fully aware of the difficulty of the case.[140]

Regarding the second aspect, the moral qualities required of a physician, Gregory saw 'humanity', or 'sympathy', as the most important one. He explained this quality and its significance as follows:

> The chief of these [moral qualities] is humanity; that sensibility of heart which makes us feel for the distresses of our fellow-creatures, and which of consequence incites us in the most powerful manner to relieve them. Sympathy produces an anxious attention to a thousand little circumstances that may tend to relieve the patient [...] Sympathy naturally engages the affection and confidence of a patient, which in many cases is of the utmost consequence to his recovery.[141]

Modern commentators, in particular bioethicist Laurence McCullough, have described the concept of sympathy, a key topic in the Scottish 'common sense' school of

---

[139] Ibid., p. 16.
[140] Ibid., pp. 17-19.
[141] Ibid., p. 19.

thought, as the cornerstone of Gregory's medical ethics. McCullough has argued that Gregory adopted his concept of sympathy from the philosopher David Hume – although there is no direct reference to Hume in the printed *Lectures* to support this claim.[142] For Gregory, sympathy was indeed the central motivating force for a doctor's moral behaviour. He acknowledged, however, that 'composure and firmness', acquired through frequently seeing scenes of distress, were also necessary for practising medicine.[143]

In addition to sympathy, Gregory called for a certain tolerance of patients' behaviours, especially their lack of compliance with strict medical instructions. While he remained paternalistic towards the patient, he advocated this tolerance (or 'indulgence' as he called it) as a matter of prudence:

---

142 Laurence B. McCullough, 'John Gregory's Medical Ethics and Humean Sympathy', in Robert Baker, Dorothy Porter and Roy Porter (eds), *The Codification of Medical Morality*, vol. 1: *Medical Ethics and Etiquette in the Eighteenth Century* (Dordrecht, Kluwer Academic Publishers, 1993), pp. 145-160. See also L. B. McCullough, *John Gregory and the Invention of Professional Medical Ethics and the Profession of Medicine* (Dordrecht, Kluwer Academic Publishers, 1998), pp. 104-114, 191-199, 214-219; idem, *John Gregory's Writings on Medical Ethics and Philosophy of Medicine* (Dordrecht, Kluwer Academic Publishers, 1998), pp. 33-39; Meinolfus Strätling, *Die Begründung der neuzeitlichen Medizinethik in Praxis, Lehre und Forschung: John Gregory (1724-1773) und seine Lectures on the Duties and Qualifications of a Physician* (Frankfurt/Main, Peter Lang, 1998), pp. 59-69. For arguments against McCullough's interpretation of Gregory's adoption of Humean sympathy, see Lisbeth Haakonssen, *Medicine and Morals in the Enlightenment: John Gregory, Thomas Percival and Benjamin Rush* (Amsterdam, Rodopi, 1997), pp. 70-74.

143 Gregory, *Lectures*, p. 20.

otherwise, patients would conceal deviations from the prescribed treatment from their physician, leading him to erroneous judgements about the course of the illness.[144] Gregory was careful, however, to preserve the physician's authority:

> This indulgence, however, which I am pleading for, must be managed with judgement and discretion; as it is very necessary that a physician should support a proper dignity and authority with his patients, for their sakes as well as his own.[145]

Patience and sympathy were, in Gregory's experience, especially required in treating people with nervous ailments. While their fears were usually 'groundless', their sufferings were 'real'.[146]

Secrecy was seen as another moral quality required of a physician, particularly as he got access to patients and their families in 'disadvantageous circumstances' and 'humiliating situations'. The reputation of patients and their families, Gregory warned his students, depended on the physician's 'discretion, secrecy, and honour'. Secrecy was thought to be especially necessary in female patients and women's conditions.[147] Further moral requirements of a physician in Gregory's view were temperance and sobriety, as intoxication impaired judgement and understanding; and candour, in

---

[144] Ibid., pp. 22-23.
[145] Ibid., p. 23.
[146] Ibid., pp. 23-24.
[147] Ibid., pp. 26-27.

the sense of being ready to acknowledge errors and rectify mistakes in treatment.[148]

Turning to the third aspect, decorum and manners, Gregory generally distinguished between those founded in 'nature and common sense', which immutably applied to all ages and nations; and those based on caprice, fashions and customs of particular nations, which were 'fluctuating and less binding'.[149] Matters discussed here by Gregory included the question of truth-telling if the patient's illness was so serious that his or her life was in danger. In this situation, Gregory believed, a deviation from the truth was justifiable (in order to preserve the patient's hope), but the patient's relatives should be informed of the real danger, especially if the patient still needed to settle his financial affairs.[150] It also gave the relatives the opportunity to call for further medical assistance if they wished.

Importantly, the physician should not abandon the dying patient, but alleviate pain and 'smooth the avenues of death, when unavoidable'.[151] This latter demand went back to Francis Bacon, who had included it in his discussion of 'euthanasia' in his *Advancement of Learning* (1605). For Bacon, one of the physician's duties was the 'euthanasia exterior', that is, the relief of terminal physical suffering 'to

[148] Ibid., pp. 27-29.
[149] Ibid., p. 32.
[150] See also chapter 2, above.
[151] Gregory, *Lectures*, pp. 34-35.

make a fayre and easie passage'.[152] This could be done at the time by giving opium preparations and alcohol, but actively shortening the patient's life was regarded as impermissible. The 'external' euthanasia, provided by the physician, was complemented by the 'euthanasia interior', i.e. the preparation of the patient's soul for the afterlife, which was traditionally the task of the clergy. When a clergyman was called in to attend to the dying patient, the physician should collaborate with him, Gregory advised. The conversation with the clergyman, he pointed out, might compose the patient's anguished mind, but he warned that 'a gloomy and indiscreet enthusiast' might harm the patient, even to the extent of shortening 'a life that otherwise might be saved'.[153] Gregory thus not only saw an important role for the physician in caring for dying patients, but also regarded him in a way as their protector against overzealous clergy.[154] Gregory furthermore defended physicians against the charge of irreligion. If a physician had 'the misfortune to disbelieve in a future state' he should conceal this sentiment from his patients.[155]

---

152 Francis Bacon, *The Advancement of Learning*, ed. by Michael Kiernan (Oxford, Clarendon Press, 2000), pp. 100-101.

153 Gregory, *Lectures*, p. 36.

154 See also Robert B. Baker and Laurence B. McCullough, 'Medical Ethics Through the Life Cycle in Europe and the Americas', in *The Cambridge World History of Medical Ethics*, ed. by R. B. Baker and L. B. McCullough (New York, Cambridge University Press, 2009), pp. 137-162, on p. 150.

155 Gregory, *Lectures*, p. 69.

Much of Gregory's deliberations on decorum and manners referred to the behaviour towards other healers, as discussed above. In addition, he commented on the issue of prescribing secret remedies or nostrums of undisclosed composition. While he acknowledged that such remedies, when new, might have a positive effect on the patient's imagination, Gregory held that they hindered the 'advancement of the art' and led to neglect of known and approved treatments.[156]

These topics were covered by Gregory in the first two of his *Lectures*, before entering a detailed description of the fourth aspect, the necessary education of a physician for successful and reputable practice, in the next three lectures. In these lectures he did not directly address matters of ethics or conduct, but discussed the educational and intellectual requirements of the physician, largely following Baconian ideals.[157] Knowledge in anatomy, physiology, natural philosophy and chemistry was regarded as fundamental. In the sixth and final lecture of this series, Gregory came back to professional ethics, arguing for the opening up of medicine to men of science, such as the Reverend Stephen Hales (who had done important experimental work on blood circulation and blood pressure, in the early eighteenth century), to

---

[156] Ibid., pp. 60-61.
[157] For discussions of Gregory's Baconianism, see Haakonssen, *Medicine and Morals*, pp. 59-62; McCullough, *John Gregory and the Invention*, pp. 187-191; Strätling, *Die Begründung*, pp. 151-159.

improve medical knowledge.[158] Gregory ended his lectures with a reflection on the dignity of the profession, which in his view was supported by medical men's commitment to learning and scientific knowledge as well as by gentlemanly behaviour:

> [...] this dignity is not supported by a narrow, selfish, corporation-spirit; by self-importance; a formality in dress and manners, or by an affectation of mystery. The true dignity of physic [i.e. medicine] is to be maintained by the superior learning and abilities of those who profess it, by the liberal manners of gentlemen, and by the openness and candour, which disdain all artifice, which invite to a free inquiry, and thus boldly bid defiance to all that illiberal ridicule and abuse to which medicine has been so much and so long exposed.[159]

Gregory thus provided an approach to medical ethics that focused on the moral psychology of the ideal physician, drawing upon the philosophical concept of sympathy and on contemporary standards of gentlemanly conduct. Moreover, his emphasis on Baconian ideas of scientific knowledge acquisition indicated that medical learning itself had for him a moral dimension, as it provided the basis for

---

[158] Gregory, *Lectures*, p. 220. See Stephen Hales, *Statical Essays: Containing Haemastaticks; or an Account of some Hydraulick and Hydrostatical Experiments made on the Blood and Blood-Vessels of Animals* (London, W. Innys and R. Manby, and T. Woodward, 1733).

[159] Gregory, *Lectures*, pp. 237-238.

rational practice to the benefit of patients. These general Enlightenment ideas were supplemented by Gregory's advice on specific aspects of medical practice, such as secrecy, truth-telling, care for the dying, behaviour towards patients more generally, and interaction with other medical practitioners, particularly during consultations. Gregory's *Lectures* were influential on other writers about medical ethics in the late eighteenth-century and beyond, especially Thomas Gisborne and Thomas Percival, to whom I will turn in the next two sections.

Gisborne: A Clergyman's Perspective on Medical Ethics

Thomas Gisborne (1758–1846), a graduate of St John's College in Cambridge, was a divine of the Church of England, serving first as perpetual curate in Yoxall (Staffordshire) and later as a prebend at Durham Cathedral. His two-volume *Enquiry into the Duties of Men in the Higher and Middle Classes of Society in Great Britain* was first published in 1794 and went through six editions, the last one appearing in 1811.[160] This wide-ranging work on professional and practical ethics covered, in volume 1, the general rights and duties of subjects and citizens, duties of the Sovereign, peers, MPs,

[160] Roy Porter, 'Thomas Gisborne: Physicians, Christians and Gentlemen', in *Doctors and Ethics: The Earlier Historical Setting of Professional Ethics*, ed. by Andrew Wear, Johanna Geyer-Kordesch and Roger French (Amsterdam, Rodopi, 1993), pp. 252-273, on pp. 254-255.

civil servants, naval and military officers, members of the legal profession, and magistrates; and in volume 2, the duties of the clerical profession, physicians, gentlemen engaged in trade and business, and of men of private means. His chapter 'On the Duties of Physicians' was, as Gisborne acknowledged, influenced by Gregory's *Lectures* and by Percival's 'Medical Jurisprudence' (i.e. the preliminary version of the later *Medical Ethics* that Percival pre-circulated among colleagues and friends).[161]

Gisborne structured the chapter in four sections, discussing (1) duties of the medical student; (2) the situation of a physician who is just beginning to practise in the profession; (3) the duties of the practising physician, subdivided into conduct towards patients, their families and friends, towards other physicians, and towards persons in the lower ranks of the medical profession; and (4) 'collateral studies and pursuits' appropriate for a physician.

For medical students the most important subjects were, in Gisborne's opinion, theory and practice of medicine, and anatomy, but they also needed to acquaint themselves sufficiently with surgery in order to be able 'to form a proper judgement' when meeting later in consultations with surgeons. Collateral subjects included chemistry, botany and

---

161 Thomas Gisborne, *An Enquiry into the Duties of Men in the Higher and Middle Classes of Society in Great Britain, Resulting from their Respective Stations, Professions, and Employments*, 2 vols, 3rd edn (London, B. and J. White, 1795), vol. 2, p. 121.

natural philosophy.[162] They should also acquire a certain degree of legal knowledge, which would help them if they needed to give evidence in court.[163] Furthermore they should not neglect 'public worship, and the private perusal and investigation of the Scriptures', and 'not be persuaded or ridiculed into drunkenness or any fashionable vice'.[164] While not directly referring here to Gregory's concept of sympathy, Gisborne warned against a hardening of feelings through frequent witnessing of dissections, operations and scenes of patient suffering:

> Let him [i.e. the medical student] beware lest his heart be rendered hard, and his deportment unfeeling, by attendance of dissections of the dead and painful operations on the living; and by being accustomed in his daily visits at an hospital to see and hear multitudes labouring in every stage and under every variety of disease.[165]

The young physician starting out in practice should avoid using improper methods of introducing himself, such as exaggerated testimonials from friends, pompousness, undermining of rivals, and servility towards powerful people. He needed to exercise temperance in eating and drinking (as physicians had to at any time of their practice), not only to be alert and in an unclouded state, but also because

---

[162] Ibid., pp. 127-128.
[163] Ibid., pp. 130-131.
[164] Ibid., pp. 132, 134.
[165] Ibid., pp. 134-135.

he could not demand such temperate behaviour from his patients if he was not serving as an example.[166]

The primary duties of the practising physician, Gisborne emphasised, were diligent and early attention to his patients.[167] Like Gregory, Gisborne demanded secrecy from the physician, especially as he got access to sensitive information in the households of his patients.[168]

However, Gisborne made an important qualification. The physician had to keep confidentiality in appropriate circumstances, but should never lie in order to do a favour to his patient:

> On proper occasions secrecy likewise is incumbent on the Physician. But he ought to promise secrecy on proper occasions alone; and he should not forget to impress on his own mind, and on that of the person who consults him, that no promise of secrecy can require or justify the telling of a falsehood.[169]

Delicacy had to be observed towards all patients, particularly female patients, and care had to be taken not to embarrass them.[170] Gisborne's rules for the general conduct of the physician towards patients were very similar to Gregory's (without citing him here):

---

[166] Ibid., pp. 137-140.
[167] Ibid., p. 141.
[168] Ibid., p. 169.
[169] Ibid., pp. 141-142.
[170] Ibid., p. 142.

> The general behaviour of the Physician towards his patient is then the most beneficial, as well as the most amiable, when he unites with the steadiness which is necessary to secure a compliance with his injunctions, those kind and gentle manners which bespeak his sympathy with the sufferer. A prudent control over the sick person and all his attendants must ever be preserved.[171]

The physician's manners, 'characterised by kindness and compassion', should enable the patient to regard him as his friend. He should exercise particular forbearance in claiming fees from patients who could ill afford them, and carefully avoid being seen as avaricious, an image physicians then had in public.[172]

The physician needed to avoid alarming patients by unguardedly discussing their case in their presence with other practitioners. However, he should not despise information from the apothecary and nurses who might be familiar with the patient's constitution by frequently attending him.[173] With reference to Percival, Gisborne advised the physician to occasionally encourage the patient that all went well, if this was consistent with the truth. Gisborne was stricter, however, than Gregory regarding truth-telling in serious illnesses, insisting that the physician was at liberty to say little, but that little had to be true. A 'mistaken tenderness'

---

[171] Ibid., pp. 142-143.
[172] Ibid., pp. 143-146.
[173] Ibid., p. 147.

must not lead him to falsehood towards the patient and their family, Gisborne warned, citing St. Paul's direction 'not to do evil that good may come'.[174] Like Gregory, Gisborne exhorted the physician not to abandon incurable patients: his continued attendance would 'compose the minds and alleviate the sorrow of friends and relations'.[175]

At the time of Gisborne's writing, physicians' consulting practice in charity hospitals had become an important feature of their work. Moreover, the training of doctors, surgeons and apothecaries increasingly included experience in hospital practice[176] Gisborne warned in this context against the temptation to make 'unnecessary or rash experiments' on poor hospital patients.[177] He was cautiously clarifying his point here, however:

> It is not meant by these remarks to censure experiments designed to lessen the danger, or the sufferings, of the individual, when founded on rational analogies; commenced after mature deliberation; conducted by upright and skilled men; watched during the whole progress with circumspect attention; and abandoned in time when unfavourable appearances take place. But it is meant to strongly reprobate every experiment rashly or

---

[174] Ibid., pp. 148-149. See also chapter 2, above.
[175] Gisborne, *Enquiry*, vol. 2, pp. 155-156.
[176] See Susan C. Lawrence, *Charitable Knowledge: Hospital Pupils and Practitioners in Eighteenth-Century London* (New York, Cambridge University Press, 1996).
[177] Gisborne, *Enquiry*, vol. 2, p. 157.

hastily adopted; or carried on by the selfish, the ignorant, the careless, or the obstinate. Proceedings of this nature are highly criminal [...].[178]

Turning to the relationships with other medical practitioners, Gisborne acknowledged that the proper behaviour of a physician to his competitors and to 'inferior members of the medical profession' was a prominent part of his duties. His conduct here should be guided by 'Christian principles' and exercised with a 'Christian temper'. With his rivals he should contend 'for public favour openly and honourably'.[179] Similarly to Gregory, Gisborne admonished the physician not to be influenced in consultations by private dislike of the other practitioner and not to look down on practitioners who had no university degree if they nevertheless had the relevant knowledge.[180]

The physician's wider social role, Gisborne suggested, could be exercised by promoting or superintending medical

---

[178] Ibid., pp. 158-159. Gisborne also advocated a restrictive use of experiments on animals: 'Neither the right nor the propriety of making these experiments on reasonable occasions can be disputed: but every degree of needless and inconsiderate cruelty in prosecuting them will be avoided with scrupulous care by men of feeling and reflection.' Ibid., p. 160. For lay and medical attitudes towards animal experiments in the eighteenth century, see Andreas-Holger Maehle, 'The Ethical Discourse on Animal Experimentation, 1650-1900', in *Doctors and Ethics: The Earlier Historical Setting of Professional Ethics*, ed. by Andrew Wear, Johanna Geyer-Kordesch and Roger French (Amsterdam, Rodopi, 1993), pp. 203-251.
[179] Gisborne, *Enquiry*, vol. 2, p. 162.
[180] Ibid., pp. 164, 166-167.

institutions such as hospitals, dispensaries and lunatic asylums, and societies for the relief of widows and orphans of deceased members of the medical profession, and by offering at a particular time of the week gratuitous treatment for the indigent poor.[181]

Other activities promoting the health of the public included advising apothecaries about new methods of treatment and new medicines and devising and making public new methods to protect the health of artisans working in 'unwholesome manufactures'.[182]

Unsurprisingly, Gisborne also commented on the charge of infidelity and irreligious behaviour that Gregory had already addressed. While Gregory had advised that the physician who did not believe in an afterlife should conceal this in the interest of his patients, Gisborne followed the line of truthfulness (as in the case of truth-telling in serious illnesses):

> This charge may have been made on partial and insufficient grounds; but the existence of it should excite the efforts of every conscientious Physician to rescue himself from the general stigma. It should stimulate him, not to affect a sense of religion which he does not entertain; but openly to avow that which he actually feels.[183]

---

[181] Ibid., pp. 174-176.
[182] Ibid., pp. 177-178.
[183] Ibid., p. 180.

Still, as far as his professional commitments, such as patient visits on Sundays, permitted, the physician should 'unite with his fellow Christians in prayers and praises to his Maker'.[184]

Gisborne's writing on medical ethics was thus characterised by his application of principles of Christian ethics, such as truthfulness and charity. He did not differ substantially from Gregory in his description of the ideal personality and behaviour of the physician (and medical student), emphasising likewise the need for sympathy, kindness and compassion, but his uncompromising commitment to veracity produced a stricter attitude when discussing medical secrecy and what the physician should say to his terminally ill patients. A new field of concern highlighted by Gisborne was the danger of abuse of poor hospital patients in medical experimentation. The restrictions that he suggested regarding human trials were similar to those that Percival outlined in his discussion of hospital practice in his *Medical Ethics,* a book that became highly influential on the codification of medical ethics in the United States of America in the nineteenth century.

---

[184] Ibid., p. 185.

Percival: Virtuous Conduct and Professional Relations

As historian of medicine John Pickstone has shown, Percival's book arose from a medico-political conflict around 1790 over an extension of the Manchester Infirmary to provide more outpatient care and home visits. In the wake of this conflict, Thomas Percival (1740–1804), who was not only a successful physician in private practice but also an 'extraordinary' consultant physician to the Infirmary, an established writer on moral matters, and an influential figure in Manchester's civic and cultural life, was asked by the hospital's physicians and surgeons to draw up rules of conduct. Having circulated a preliminary version, entitled 'Medical Jurisprudence', to colleagues and friends in 1794, Percival expanded his work to cover medical ethics beyond the hospital setting.

By the time of its publication in 1803, one year before his death, Percival's *Medical Ethics* was, as Pickstone has suggested, a belated defence of virtuous medical behaviour rooted in a past Enlightenment social order which was then threatened by industrialisation, urbanisation, and repressive politics in reaction to the French revolution.[185]

Nevertheless, Percival's text served as a blueprint for the ethical codes of newly formed medical societies in nineteenth-century America, particularly that of the American Medical Association in 1847, perpetuating through this route a conservative ideal of the virtuous and responsible doctor. Writing in an aphoristic style, Percival covered, in four chapters professional conduct (1) in hospitals and other medical charities such as dispensaries, lock hospitals for venereal diseases, and mental institutions; (2) in private or general practice; (3) in the relationship of physicians to apothecaries; and (4) in cases which touched upon the law. An appendix of 'Notes and Illustrations' elaborated on his thinking about specific ethical matters.[186]

Two overarching themes are recognisable in Percival's rules for hospital practice: to maximize the benefit to the mostly poor charity patients in the voluntary hospitals and other charitable institutions of his time; and to facilitate co-operation between the physicians and surgeons who held honorary appointments to these institutions in addition to

---

[185] John V. Pickstone, 'Thomas Percival and the Production of Medical Ethics', in Robert Baker, Dorothy Porter and Roy Porter (eds), *The Codification of Medical Morality*, vol. 1: *Medical Ethics and Etiquette in the Eighteenth Century* (Dordrecht, Kluwer Academic Publishers, 1993), pp. 161-178. See also Robert Baker, 'Deciphering Percival's Code', ibid., pp. 179-211; Haakonssen, *Medicine and Morals*, pp. 94-186.

[186] The following references are to the Oxford 1849 edition, *Percival's Medical Ethics* (Reprint Leopold Classic Library).

their private practices. At the very start of these deliberations, he reminded his medical readers of their serious responsibility for the health and life of the sick admitted to the institution, to treat them with 'tenderness' as well as with 'steadiness' and with 'condescension' (in the contemporary sense of treating them as if they were socially equals) as well as with 'authority'.[187] These basic attitudes were obviously derived from Gregory's notions of sympathetic as well as effective physician behaviour in private practice (see above), adapted by Percival to the hospital situation of treating lower class charity patients.[188] Being bound to a tacit contract between profession and society, as bioethicist Robert Baker has argued in his analysis of Percival's text, hospital practitioners were supposed to protect the interests of the charity patients, e.g. against too strict parsimony of the infirmary's board of trustees in supplying high-quality medicines.[189]

Percival emphasised the need to consider hospital patients' emotions, and to treat them respectfully, highlighting especially the vulnerability of female patients, and – in a special section on lunatic asylums – of the mentally ill.[190] Secrecy had to be observed where circumstances required it, and care had to be taken that conversations with the patient

[187] Ibid., p. 27.
[188] See also Baker, 'Deciphering Percival's Code', pp. 194-195.
[189] Ibid., pp. 199-200; *Percival's Medical Ethics,* pp. 30-31.
[190] Ibid., pp.28-29, 42, 45.

were not overheard by others in the large wards of the infirmary.[191] Percival was generally in favour of trying new remedies or new surgical procedures on hospital patients for the public good, and especially in the interest of the poor as the largest section of society, when no conventional treatment had helped. He thus seemed to imply that such experimentation could be justified as serving the poor hospital patients' own interests, or at least those of their class, as well as public interests at large. Like Gisborne he indicated, however, his awareness of the danger of abuse, demanding that a new method of treatment should be based on 'sound reason, just analogy, or well authenticated facts' and that no trial should be started before a consultation among the relevant physicians or surgeons had taken place.[192] His concern for hospital patients was paternalistic. For example, discussion of the patient's condition with other practitioners or students should not happen in the presence of the patient to avoid misapprehension and fears; and the difficulty or danger of an illness requiring consultations between the hospital's physicians and surgeons should be concealed from the patient to avoid 'anxiety and alarm'.[193]

Rules for consultations were also a major concern for Percival in order to achieve smooth collaboration between surgeons and physicians. Here his advice was supporting

---

[191] Ibid., p. 29.

[192] Ibid., p. 32.

[193] Ibid., pp. 28-29, 38. See also chapter 2, above.

the contemporary hierarchical relationship between the two professional groups. The most junior practitioner should first venture an opinion, the consultation then going upwards to the most senior practitioner (who would thus have the last word), with the most junior physician speaking after the most senior surgeon. Percival advocated, however, joint, majority decisions about the treatment plan for the patient, and if such a decision could not be reached, the surgeon or physician in charge of the hospital patient concerned was supposed to determine how to proceed further. Obviously being conscious of the sensitive nature of these consultation rules, Percival added that they had originally been suggested to him by a physician and a surgeon, Dr John Ferriar and Mr William Simmons, both from Manchester.[194] More generally, Percival sought to contain professional conflict within the institution, urging to find internal solutions in order to avoid reputational damage for the profession in the eyes of the public.[195]

Percival's discussion of professional conduct in private practice opened with the assertion that the core requirements of treating patients with 'attention, steadiness, and humanity' applied here as well, as did the need for secrecy, discretion and delicacy.[196] This statement was not surpris-

---

[194] *Percival's Medical Ethics,* pp. 36-39.
[195] Ibid., pp. 31-32.
[196] Ibid., p. 47.

ing, given that he had in several of his recommendations regarding hospital patients tried to make their situation as similar as possible to the more privileged position of the usually middle-class, or upper-class, patients of private practice outside of the institution. Other requirements of private practice, according to Percival, included temperance, in order to be in an unclouded state when practising, and avoidance of gloomy prognostications, as they smacked of empiricism by unduly magnifying the importance of the physician's treatment, and in order to preserve the patient's hope (see also chapter 2 above).[197]

Much of Percival's further advice aimed at avoiding friction with other practitioners: not to interfere with a colleague's treatment of a patient, unless there was clear evidence that it endangered the patient's life; to justify a colleague's treatment as far as this was consistent with the truth; to stick to one's role as either physician or surgeon, at least in towns with a relatively high number of practitioners; and to be open-minded and courteous during consultations with other practitioners, observing seniority as in hospital practice, the seniority here being determined by the time a physician or surgeon had practised in the place of his residence.[198] Discussions between the consulting practitioners should not be held in front of patients or relatives, and only prognoses which had been previously agreed upon

[197] Ibid., pp. 47-49.
[198] Ibid., pp. 49-54, 63.

should be issued.[199] Like Gregory, Percival regarded it as a moral duty to attend to and not to abandon dying patients.[200]

Percival advocated local agreements between practitioners about the level of fees to be charged, while maintaining some flexibility to require more from affluent patients and less from those in need. Colleagues and their families should usually be treated for free.[201] Other rules concerned accuracy and truthfulness in issuing sick notes, not to prescribe patent remedies of unknown composition, and to keep intra-professional disputes away from the public, again to protect the profession's reputation.[202] Like Gregory and Gisborne, Percival urged medical practitioners to attend church services, seeing religion also as a force to counteract the development of a hardened, unsympathetic attitude through long practice.[203] Being himself in his early sixties, Percival finally exhorted aging colleagues to be self-critical about their remaining abilities, to accept with good grace consultations with younger colleagues if so wished by the patient, and to retire in time as a professional duty to society when one's capacities had declined too far.[204]

---

[199] Ibid., pp. 54-55,
[200] Ibid., p. 55.
[201] Ibid., pp. 56-58, 62.
[202] Ibid., pp. 59-62.
[203] Ibid., pp. 65, 160-161.
[204] Ibid., pp. 65-68.

Many of Percival's rules concerning professional relations were due to considerable overlaps between the patientcare then provided by physicians, surgeons and apothecaries, especially in provincial England.[205] Percival devoted a special chapter to the conduct of physicians towards apothecaries, as he perceived a particularly close connection between these two professional groups.[206] A physician's success and reputation, he argued, depended to a large extent on the 'knowledge, skill and fidelity' of the apothecary, who was usually the physician's precursor in treating a case. During the subsequent treatment the physician should cooperate with the apothecary to their mutual reputational benefit as well as in the interest of the patient.[207] Such cooperation should, however, as Percival emphasised, not prevent the physician from carrying out occasional, semi-official quality controls of the drugs and medicines kept in the apothecary's shop.[208] The hierarchy between the two groups was also reflected in Percival's advice to physicians to refuse patients' requests to act as temporary substitutes if the apothecary was absent. The honour of the profession demanded that a physician could only be

---

[205] See Michael Brown, *Performing medicine: Medical culture and identity in provincial England, c. 1760-1850* (Manchester and New York, Manchester University Press, 2011), pp. 17-18.

[206] For a contemporary example of such close connections, see Brown's discussion of York apothecary Oswald Allen and physician (and Allen's brother-in-law) Dr Thomas Withers, ibid., pp. 32-39.

[207] *Percival's Medical Ethics*, pp. 69-71.

[208] Ibid., pp. 71-72.

substituting for another physician, a surgeon for a surgeon, and an apothecary for an apothecary.[209] In preserving the professional distinctions Percival aimed at avoiding conflicts through overlaps in practice, similarly as he did in his chapters on hospital and private practice.

Percival's fourth and final chapter in *Medical Ethics* dealt with a variety of professional duties under the existing law. Covering topics such as assessments of mental capacity for last wills or for commitments to a lunatic asylum, and physicians' and surgeons' testimony in coroner's inquests and in trials for murder or rape, he stressed the need for very careful consideration of the evidence in each case, given the serious consequences which medical expert statements could have.[210] While Percival acknowledged that such medico-legal duties were inconvenient for practitioners, he insisted on their fulfilment as a debt to the community.[211] A matter of special concern to him was the role of medical practitioners in attending duels, which in his opinion might make them as guilty as those who acted as seconds in a duel.[212]

In his comments on abortion, Percival noted that the giving of abortifacient drugs was not always unlawful: it could be justified if a too narrow pelvis of the pregnant woman

---

[209] Ibid., pp. 74-75.
[210] Ibid., pp. 81-84, 87-88, 109-117.
[211] Ibid., p.120.
[212] Ibid., pp. 102-109.

would make birth impossible and fatal. Otherwise, however, he equated abortion with the murder of a child.[213] He also discussed the social problem of infanticide, largely sharing here the sympathetic view of the eminent London obstetrician William Hunter (1718-1783), who had emphasised the emotional distress and sense of shame of women who had secretly given birth to a child out of wedlock. Percival regarded the then existing death penalty for infanticide as too harsh and hoped for a revision of the law.[214] In general terms, however, he reminded his colleagues of their legal obligation to state the whole truth and not to leave out any relevant facts when giving testimony in court, even if this might lead to capital punishment of the accused.[215]

Percival's *Medical Ethics* thus provided a comprehensive account of desirable medical conduct, in relation to patients, society at large, and the various interactions of the then three professional groups, physicians, surgeons, and apothecaries.[216] The different dimensions of professional ethics were interlinked, for example in the issue of consultations, which were supposed to happen without friction between the practitioners involved in the best interest of the patient. Subsequent writers on medical ethics in the nineteenth century drew heavily on Percival's aphoristic text, elaborating

---

[213] Ibid., pp. 94-95. On the issue of abortion, see chapter 5, below.

[214] *Percival's Medical Ethics*, pp. 96-101.

[215] Ibid., pp. 122-124.

[216] See also Gary S. Belkin, 'History and Bioethics: The Uses of Thomas Percival', *Medical Humanities Review* 12 (1998), pp. 39-59.

on it in some points and adapting it to changing social and political circumstances.

The Legacy of Percival: Ryan, the AMA Code, and Styrap

One such writer was the Irish physician Michael Ryan (1794–1840), who practised in London and taught medicine, obstetrics and medical jurisprudence at several of its private medical schools.[217] Ryan, who belonged to the medical reformers of his day, deplored that the teaching of professional ethics to medical students was 'almost totally neglected' and that the moral statutes and obligations required by some of the Royal Colleges were so few and little known that they were 'nearly useless'.[218] His *Manual of Medical Jurisprudence* (second edition 1836, first published 1831) therefore included a substantial part on medical ethics, from 'Hippocrates' to the 'Present Age'. In this latter chapter he reproduced much of Percival's *Medical Ethics* and gave a summary of Gregory's *Lectures*, adding his personal

[217] For a biographical account of Ryan see Howard Brody, Zahra Meghani and Kimberley Greenwald (eds), *Michael Ryan's Writings on Medical Ethics* (Dordrecht, Springer, 2010), pp. 17-34.

[218] Michael Ryan, 'A Manual of Medical Jurisprudence, and State Medicine' (2nd edition 1836), reprinted in Brody, Meghani and Greenwald, *Michael Ryan's Writings on Medical Ethics*, pp. 79-222, on p. 141. On the medical reform movement of the early nineteenth century, see Adrian J. Desmond, *The Politics of Evolution: Morphology, Medicine and Reform* (Chicago, University of Chicago Press, 1989); Roger French and Andrew Wear (eds), *British Medicine in an Age of Reform* (London, Routledge, 1991).

comments. He also cited the brief 1835 *Statutes of Morality* of the Royal College of Physicians of London, which specified penalties for misconduct in inter-practitioner relations, such as unjustified accusations of ignorance or malpractice, poaching another practitioner's patients, making underhand deals with apothecaries on prescription fees, and failing to observe the rules on consultations.[219]

Ryan's remarks on medical confidentiality and on truth-telling in serious illness, which largely followed Percival's advice on these topics, have already been mentioned above (see chapters 1 and 2). Some differences to Percival emerged in Ryan's assessment of the ethics of experimenting on patients. He addressed this issue within his comments on the medical oath of the University of Edinburgh, which demanded that medical men must practise 'cautiously, chastely, and honourably'.[220] For Ryan, cautious practice meant to use or recommend only those treatments that one would apply to oneself or one's own family members in the same situation, following the Golden Rule, 'Do unto others as you would they should do unto you'.[221] He acknowledged that trying out new remedies was a necessity in medicine in the interest of the patients concerned if no other

---

[219] Ryan, 'Manual of Medical Jurisprudence', pp. 153-154.
[220] For an analysis of the Edinburgh medical oath, which dates back to 1732, see Robert Baker, *Before Bioethics: A History of American Medical Ethics from the Colonial Period to the Bioethics Revolution* (New York, Oxford University Press, 2013), pp. 43-52.
[221] Ryan, 'Manual of Medical Jurisprudence', p. 156. Cf. Matthew 7:12.

treatments were known. But Ryan sharply condemned any doctor administering 'a dangerous medicine, merely to gratify his own curiosity, or zeal for science – to ascertain the comparative advantage or disadvantage of some new remedy'. Such conduct would constitute 'a high misdemeanour, and a great breach of trust towards his patient'.[222] Instead, he pointed to the options of experimenting on animals, or – again in line with the Golden Rule – of self-experiments by medical men.[223] Thus, Ryan took a considerably stricter line on clinical experimentation than Percival had done.

Furthermore, as an obstetric physician, he was particularly explicit about the need for strict moral conduct in examining female patients – a topic that Gregory and Percival had only hinted at. The patient's mother or other near relative, or an intimate female friend, should be present, and the doctor should in his examination of the woman's body conduct himself in such a way as to avoid any later accusations of a 'slipper hand' or 'impure mind'.[224] Ryan discussed more specific ethical issues of obstetric practice in another work, his *Manual of Midwifery,* to which I will turn in the next chapter.

---

[222] Ryan, 'Manual of Medical Jurisprudence', pp. 156-157.
[223] Ibid., p. 157.
[224] Ibid., p. 158.

Percival's legacy continued, as mentioned, through the adoption of many of his rules by the newly founded American Medical Association in its 1847 *Code of Ethics*. Yet, while the AMA code largely followed Percival's ethics, its structure and its emphasis on certain issues responded to different social circumstances for American doctors. As modern commentators such as Robert Baker and Stanley Joel Reiser have pointed out, the American code adapted Percival's hierarchical perspective on the medical profession to a more egalitarian social environment. In particular, the AMA code was written by a group of regular physicians to define standards of conduct that would demarcate them from irregular healers or 'quacks' and from 'sectarian' practitioners such as the homeopaths.[225] It was thus a document which aimed not only at medical practitioners, but also intended to convince patients and the public at large that the 'regulars', i.e. those trained at established medical schools, were the healers who deserved their trust and respect.

This intention was reflected in the structuring of the AMA code into three chapters, each of which dealt with *reciprocal* duties: between physicians and their patients; mu-

[225] See Robert Baker, 'The Historical Context of the American Medical Association's 1847 *Code of Ethics*', in R. Baker (ed.), *The Codification of Medical Morality*, vol. 2: *Anglo-American Medical Ethics and Medical Jurisprudence in the Nineteenth Century* (Dordrecht, Kluwer Academic Publishers, 1995), pp. 47-63; Stanley Joel Reiser, 'Creating a Medical Profession in the United States: The First Code of Ethics of the American Medical Association', ibid., pp. 89-103.

tually between physicians and their profession; and between the profession and the public. Compared to Percival's *Medical Ethics*, doctors' duties in the AMA code did not differ very much, including matters such as confidentiality, restricted truth-telling in serious illness, care for the dying, and the observation of various rules for consultations with other practitioners.[226] The latter rules demanded though that only those with a regular, scientific medical education were acceptable for consultation and excluded the adherents of 'an exclusive dogma' (e.g. homeopaths).[227] New was also the prohibition of any form of medical advertising, whether through cards or handbills or through publishing about cases and operations in the daily press. Such conduct, typically linked to irregular forms of practice in a commercial environment, was thought to be 'derogatory to the dignity of the profession'.[228]

Significantly, the number of stipulated obligations of patients to their physicians exceeded the physicians' duties to their patients and included as 'first duty' the selection of a medical adviser who had 'received a regular professional education'. Other patient duties included sticking to only one physician as far as possible, and to ask for a consultation only with the consent of the currently attending physician; to present with symptoms at an early stage; to be truthful

---

[226] Isaac Hays, 'Code of Ethics', ibid., pp. 75-87.
[227] Ibid., p. 81.
[228] Ibid., p. 80.

about possible causes of an illness; to comply with prescriptions; to pay fees promptly; and if wanting to change physician, to give the current one an explanation for it.[229] Such rules specifically reflected the competitive climate in which many American doctors practised in the first half of the nineteenth century. With a number of changes these rules were adopted in the 1870s for a British code of medical ethics, compiled by the English physician Jukes Styrap (1815–1899).

As Styrap noted in the preface to his *A Code of Medical Ethics* (first published 1878, subsequent editions 1886, 1890, 1895), he had used the regulations of the Manchester and Salopian Medico-Ethical Societies and especially the 1847 code of ethics of the American Medical Association, which in turn were based on Percival's text.[230] In contrast to the AMA, however, there was a strand of opinion in the British medical profession, including the British Medical Association, that medical ethics did not require an explicit, written code. Two BMA select committees given the task to devise a code of ethics in the 1840s and 1850s had failed to meet;[231] and when in 1882 Styrap offered his code to the BMA, a

---

[229] Ibid., pp. 77-79.

[230] Jukes Styrap, *A Code of Medical Ethics: With Remarks on the Duties of Practitioners to Their Patients; and the Obligations of Patients to Their Medical Advisers: Also on the Duties of the Profession to the Public, and the Obligations of the Public to the Faculty* (London, J. & A. Churchill, 1878), p. 3.

[231] Ibid.; Peter Bartrip, 'An Introduction to Jukes Styrap's *A Code of Medical Ethics* (1878)', in Baker, *Codification of Medical Morality*, vol. 2, pp. 145-148, on p. 146.

copy to be sent to every new member, the Association's Committee of Council politely declined, thanking him for having spent so much time and money on it, but not seeing 'their way to accept his offer.'[232] Still, by 1896 the *British Medical Journal* characterised Styrap's code as 'at present the usually accepted authority', yet also reported a resolution of the BMA's general meeting of that year to invite the Council to prepare a different, new code.[233]

Styrap had used for his code the same three-chapter structure as the authors of the AMA code, discussing the reciprocal obligations in the doctor–patient, intra-professional, and profession–public relationships. His introductory remarks showed that he was especially concerned about professional rivalries and lack of solidarity among doctors, which, he believed, harmed the profession's public reputation. Frequent social gatherings of doctors, to discuss not only scientific matters but also topics such as standards of medical education and medical ethics, were in his view a way to overcome this problem.[234] In fact, during the 1850s Styrap had served as secretary to the Salopian Medico-Ethical Society, which he had helped found, and after this society's merger with the Shropshire branch of the BMA he had

---

[232] *British Medical Journal*, July 29, 1882, p. 192.

[233] *British Medical Journal*, August 15, 1896, p. 401. See also Bartrip, 'An Introduction', p. 145. The request to the BMA Council to prepare a code of ethics does not seem to have been followed up, but in 1902, Robert Saundby, the founding chairman of the BMA's Central Ethical Committee, published the first edition of his guidebook to medical ethics. See this chapter, below.

[234] Styrap, *Code*, pp. 6-10, 17-18.

become honorary secretary.[235] Addressing the objection to a medical ethics code that 'no laws, however stringent, will make a man honourable who is not innately inclined to be so', he claimed a salutary effect of members of the profession who set a good example. Taking a more pragmatic stance, Styrap further recommended that an ethical committee or council of doctors should be founded in every county, so that cases of misconduct would be brought to the wider attention of the district's practitioners and, if necessary, of the profession at large. The attention of their colleagues would not fail to have its effect on the offending practitioners.[236] While Styrap did not mention it here, such local ethical committees might also report misbehaving practitioners to the General Medical Council, which, founded in 1858, had by the time of his writing been exercising its disciplinary function for twenty years.[237]

Although Styrap largely followed the AMA code, respectively Percival's ethics, he made some significant changes for his code, which indicated a morally stricter attitude, both towards patients and within the profession. For example, while generally requiring medical confidentiality, he stipulated exceptions in cases of 'threatening insanity' or of 'pertinacious concealment of pregnancy after seduction',

---

[235] Bartrip, 'Introduction', pp. 146-147.
[236] Styrap, *Code*, pp. 19-20.
[237] See chapter 1, above.

where a close relative of the patient should be informed.[238] Furthermore, although Styrap subscribed to the rule not to abandon incurable patients, he specified circumstances under which a doctor would be justified in relinquishing a patient's care, 'such as wilful, persistent disregard of his advice; the abuse of his attendance as a "blind" for some unworthy purpose, or irregularity of life; loss of the necessary professional restraining influence; and other positions which the practitioner's innate feeling of self-respect will at once indicate, should the necessity arise'.[239] In a similar vein, he praised the medical profession's devotion to the needs of a 'too often, selfish public', demanding almost religious respect of the patient for the physician 'for the Lord hath created him'.[240] Similar to the AMA code, Styrap expected from the public to seek advice only from scientifically educated (and, in Britain, GMC 'registered') practitioners.[241] Reflecting the recent public debates around the British *Cruelty to Animals Act* of 1876, he added under the heading 'Obligations of the Public to the Profession' a strongly worded defence of animal experimentation as a means to practical and theoretical progress in medicine, against 'the denunciatory

[238] Styrap, *Code*, p. 21.
[239] Ibid., pp. 22-23.
[240] Ibid, pp. 23-24, with reference to *Ecclus*, ch. 38.
[241] Ibid., p. 24.

and unreasonable clamour of a small, morbid section of society'.[242] Regarding disputes between medical practitioners he advocated, like Percival and the AMA had done, discreet arbitration without the patient's knowledge and away from the public eye, but he claimed that there were some practitioners who could 'only be effectively influenced by public censure', which in these cases would constitute 'a perfectly legitimate *dernier ressort* through the action of a "Court Medical"'.[243]

Brudenell Carter: Explaining Medical Ethics to the Public and to the Profession

While Styrap's code of 1878 went through three further editions until the end of the nineteenth century, its moralising and sometimes harsh tone is unlikely to have endeared it beyond professional circles to a wider, more general readership. Despite the professional self-confidence that Styrap's writing reflected, there was also a perceived need in the late nineteenth-century medical profession to explain its ethics to wider audiences. This task was prominently taken on by the eye surgeon Robert Brudenell Carter (1828–

[242] Styrap, *Code*, p. 44. On the nineteenth-century anti-vivisection movement, see Nicolaas A. Rupke (ed.), *Vivisection in Historical Perspective* (London, Routledge, 1990); Rob Boddice, *The Science of Sympathy: Morality, Evolution, and Victorian Civilization* (Urbana, University of Illinois Press, 2016), pp. 53-100.
[243] Styrap, *Code*, pp. 38-40.

1918), FRCS, a consultant at St. George's Hospital, London. Brudenell Carter was a prolific medical writer, not only in ophthalmology, but also as a regular contributor and correspondent to the *Times* and the *Lancet*. From 1887 to 1899 he was the representative of the Society of Apothecaries on the General Medical Council, where he successfully introduced the practice of postponing decisions on merely minor disciplinary offences to the subsequent year, creating in this way a kind of probation period for the offending practitioner (so that the severe sanction of erasure from the Register might be avoided).[244] Brudenell Carter was thus well placed to write about medical ethics: from his experience in the GMC's professional discipline proceedings and in writing for lay as well as professional readers.

In 1899, Brudenell Carter contributed the chapter on the medical profession to a volume entitled *Unwritten Laws and Ideals of Active Careers*, edited by E. H. Pitcairn. The concept of this volume was similar to that of Gisborne's *Enquiry into the Duties of Men* a hundred years earlier in that it covered organisation, values, ethics and etiquette of a wide range of professional occupations, including politics and diplomacy, the military, the clergy, law, education, banking, architecture, and art and music, in addition to medicine.[245] Carter

---

[244] 'Obituary. R. Brudenell Carter, F.R.C.S.', *British Medical Journal*, November 2, 1918; 'Robert Brudenell Carter, F.R.C.S.', *The Lancet*, November 2, 1918.
[245] Robert Brudenell Carter, 'The Medical Profession', in E. H. Pitcairn (ed.), *Unwritten Laws and Ideals of Active Careers* (London, Smith, Elder, & Co, 1899), pp. 203-252.

started his exposition with the problem that patients and their relatives tended to regard the rules of 'medical etiquette' as a hindrance to their 'freedom of action'. In his view this was a misconception, as such rules worked 'altogether to the advantage of the community'.[246] Carter took much care to explain the institutional development of medical qualifications in the United Kingdom, describing in particular the roles of the London-based corporations, i.e. the Royal College of Physicians, Royal College of Surgeons, and the Society of Apothecaries. Moreover, he highlighted the function of the General Medical Council in safeguarding standards of medical training and examinations and in exercising professional discipline.[247]

Having addressed the by then classical issue of consultations, and having urged 'mutual respect', in the patient's interest, between attending general practitioners and (specialist) consultants, Carter made rather scathing remarks about patients who habitually sought the opinion of several doctors, either trying to conceal or distorting earlier advice received. His advice to doctors 'against people of this class' was to contact the other practitioners concerned and to 'seek friendly explanations' about the case.[248] A practitioner

---

[246] Ibid., p. 203.

[247] Ibid., pp. 204-221. One the disciplinary role of the GMC, see chapter 1, above.

[248] Brudenell Carter 'Medical Profession', pp. 224-225, 228-229, 241-242.

should not take on a colleague's case unless he had been assured that the patient had informed the colleague about the wish to change their doctor.[249] Generally, Carter encouraged, however, practitioners and patients to seek the view of a consultant in genuinely difficult and uncertain conditions. Like Percival and other previous writers, he thought though that patients should not be fully informed about the nature of their problem, in order to avoid anxiety and further complications.[250] Consultations with homeopaths or with quack doctors were strictly rejected by him, as he saw no common ground with them.[251]

Carter especially emphasised the requirement of medical confidentiality, for which he recognised only three exceptions: the legal duty of medical practitioners to give evidence about patient details as a witness in a court of law; the information of parents or guardians about the illness of a child; and legally required notification of certain infectious diseases to the public health authorities.[252] A reciprocal obligation of patients was to follow the advice of their doctor,

---

[249] Ibid., p. 248.

[250] Ibid., pp. 233-236.

[251] Ibid., pp. 242-243.

[252] Ibid., pp. 244-247. On the lack of a medical privilege in court and other confidentially issues for British medical practitioners around 1900, see Angus Ferguson, *Should a Doctor Tell? The Evolution of Medical Confidentiality in Britain* (Farnham, Ashgate, 2013); Andreas-Holger Maehle, *Contesting Medical Confidentiality: Origins of the Debate in the United States, Britain, and Germany* (Chicago, The University of Chicago Press, 2016); and chapter 5, below.

or, if this did not seem possible, to be open about the obstacles.[253] Carter concluded his discussion by stressing that medical practice was a skill, based on scientific facts and truthfulness, earning its owner a living, whereas a tradesman might make false representations about his merchandise in order to maximise his profit. Moreover, the relations between tradesmen and their customers were impersonal, whereas those between (medical) professionals and their clients (patients) were personal. Referring to the Golden Rule, he expected medical professionals to do as they would want to be done by, and hoped, in return, for the public's 'gratitude' for their services.[254]

In addition to this book chapter, Carter disseminated his views on medical ethics to further audiences, reiterating, and elaborating on, the issues mentioned above. In 1900 he published an article in the philosophical periodical *International Journal of Ethics* (the precursor of the present journal *Ethics*), in which he focused on the disciplinary function of the General Medical Council and the options of the medical colleges and societies to discipline or expel members for misconduct.[255] He admitted that the various codes of medical ethics had not been particularly successful, but acknowledged the intention of many of their clauses to mitigate

---

[253] Brudenell Carter, 'Medical Profession', pp. 247-248.

[254] Ibid., pp. 249-252.

[255] Robert Brudenell Carter, 'Medical Ethics', *International Journal of Ethics* 11/1 (1900), pp. 22-46.

competition between practitioners and to prevent 'underhand dealing' in regard to patient care. The codes, he also claimed, responded to a public interest in trustworthy and honourable practitioners.[256] He was critical, however, of intra-professional rules which, to him, had a 'trades-union spirit', and he feared that in recent years a 'decadence' from the 'standards of a man of honor to the standards of a man of business' had set in.[257]

By 1903 Carter had expanded his discussion to a book for the general reader, entitled *Doctors and Their Work*.[258] As he pointed out in its preface, he hoped to achieve 'a better understanding of medical objects and methods' and 'to show patients in what way they may best co-operate with their physicians'.[259] He provided in his book wide-ranging information on the contemporary medical profession, from education, practice and the demarcation from quackery, to medical science, specialisms, medical confidentiality, and female doctors, noting that about 300 to 400 women were by then on the Medical Register.[260] What he advocated, however, was a traditional, paternalist model of the doctor–patient relationship in which the patient was to follow the medical instructions without seeking explanations:

---

[256] Ibid., pp. 29-35.

[257] Ibid., pp. 34, 39, 45.

[258] Robert Brudenell Carter, *Doctors and Their Work or Medicine, Quackery, and Disease* (London, Smith, Elder, & Co., 1903).

[259] Ibid., p. vi.

[260] Ibid., p. 313.

> The patient whose chief desire it is to recover from his malady, and who, as a means of attaining that primary object, desires to do all that is within his power to contribute towards its attainment, will usually act wisely if he abstain from endeavours to seek popular explanations of physiological doctrine, and is content to submit himself resignedly into the hands of the doctor whom he has selected, and in whom he has confidence, and to do and avoid what he is told to do or to avoid, without disturbing his mind as regards either nomenclature or causes. His doctor will analyse his state more easily, and will ascertain it more exactly, if he is relieved from the burden of trying to find descriptive words intelligible to the non-medical mind.[261]

Whether Brudenell Carter's literary efforts made any significant impact on the doctor–patient relations of his day is questionable. But they indicate that medical ethics had developed to a degree that seemed to require detailed exposition of its rules to patients and the public more generally, as well as to incoming new doctors and fellow practitioners.

Saundby: Ethics Guidance for Medical Practitioners

Responding to pressures on medical practitioners caused by overcrowding of the profession, the provision of free care

[261] Ibid., pp. 150-151.

by outpatient departments of voluntary hospitals, and the negotiating powers of health insurance organisations for workers and artisans (the so-called Friendly Societies) when contracting with doctors, the BMA founded in 1902 a Central Ethical Committee (CEC). A structural reform of the BMA at this time involved the creation of local Divisions which were meant to serve as 'courts of honour', similar to what Styrap had envisaged in the late 1870s. The CEC was tasked to advise the Divisions, to take on matters that could not be resolved at a lower level (including cases for expulsion from the Association), and to draw up rules for dealing with difficult issues.[262] Its first chairman was Robert Saundby, professor of medicine at the University of Birmingham, who in the same year published his guidebook on medical ethics.[263] By 1907, this guide appeared in an enlarged second edition (partly because a fire at the publishers had destroyed stocks of the first edition) and constituted the most detailed British code of medical ethics published so far.[264] Saundby, then Vice President of the BMA and a Mem-

---

[262] Andrew A. G. Morrice, '"Honour and Interests": Medical Ethics and the British Medical Association', in Andreas-Holger Maehle and Johanna Geyer-Kordesch (eds), *Historical and Philosophical Perspectives on Biomedical Ethics: From Paternalism to Autonomy?* (Aldershot, Ashgate, 2002), pp. 11-35, on pp. 17-19.

[263] Robert Saundby, *Medical Ethics: A Guide to Professional Conduct* (Bristol, John Wright and Co., 1902).

[264] Robert Saundby, *Medical Ethics: A Guide to Professional Conduct*, 2nd edn, Enlarged and Rewritten (London, Charles Griffin & Company, 1907).

ber of the General Medical Council, applied his practical experience with issues of professional conduct to his writing about medical ethics. With the exception of medical confidentiality, the CEC was mostly concerned with predominantly intra-professional issues, such as solidarity among local practitioners in pay disputes with the health insurance providers, rules for consultations, and medical advertising.[265] While reflecting these prominent matters, Saundby's guidebook *Medical Ethics* followed, however, a broader conception as a reference work, succinctly discussing in alphabetical order 62 topics which ranged from 'Advertising' and 'Etiquette', via 'Midwifery' and 'Patients', to 'Surgery' and the 'Workmen's Compensation Acts'. Saundby claimed in the introduction to his work that medical ethics was built on three principles:

> In the relation of a medical practitioner towards his colleagues, he should obey the golden rule, which teaches that, 'Whatever ye would that men should do to you, do ye even so to them' (*St. Matthew*, vii. 12); in his relations to his patients, their interests should be his highest considerations – 'Aegroti salus suprema lex'; in his relation to the State, to the laws of the country, and his civic duties, there is no better guiding principle than the words of the Gospel, 'Render, therefore, unto Caesar the things

[265] See Morrice, '"Honour and Interests"', pp. 20-27.

that be Caesar's' (*St. Luke*, xx. 25); in other words, obey all lawful authority.[266]

In his advice on specific topics, however, Saundby did not provide deep thoughts based on these moral and religious principles, but largely followed the Percival–AMA–Styrap tradition of professional ethics. His rules were guided, as had been those of his predecessors, by notions of honourable and gentlemanly behaviour. In addition, he referred to resolutions of the BMA and regulations of the General Medical Council and the medical corporations. Yet, Saundby did also address a number of areas of potential moral conflict, especially in the relations to patients.

For example, reflecting on the accusation that the medical profession experimented on patients, he demanded that new treatments should only be tried out when no reliable remedy was known. If an experiment was to be conducted for the sake of gaining new knowledge, not specifically for the benefit of the patient concerned, and if it carried some risk, it required the patient's prior 'knowledge and consent'. Saundby conceded that this rule would mean slow progress in medicine and that the testing of some new methods, from hypnotic suggestion therapy to treatments with X-rays and high-frequency currents, might have been hindered by English conservatism. He defended this conservatism, however, by pointing to alleged overuse of certain methods in other

[266] Saundby, *Medical Ethics* (1907), p. 1.

countries, such as the application of the stomach pump in Germany, too frequent operations for appendicitis in the USA, and frequent gastroenterostomy operations in Italy and France.[267]

Furthermore, Saundby addressed, albeit relatively briefly, moral issues at the beginning and end of life. While noting, with approval, that abortion had been criminalised in 'all civilised and Christian countries', he raised the question in which circumstances the intervention, carried out by doctors, might still be morally and legally justified. Abortion in the interest of the 'health of the mother' was in his opinion a too liberal criterion, as it would permit the termination of almost any inopportune pregnancy. Saundby took the more conservative stance to induce premature labour only if – following confirmation by a second medical opinion – the *life* of the mother was judged to be in grave danger. If the foetus was viable, an 'operation' that could save both lives, i.e. Caesarean section, should be chosen.[268] In general, he demanded that no operation should be performed on a patient 'unless its nature, risks, and consequences have been fully explained, if not to the patient, at least to the patient's friends.'[269]

---

[267] Ibid., pp. 82, 96-97.

[268] Ibid., pp. 64, 123. On the debate about craniotomy versus Caesarean section, see chapter 4, below.

[269] Saundby, *Medical Ethics* (1902), p. 56.

Saundby likewise followed a cautious, conservative line in the question of euthanasia, which he defined as 'the doctrine that it is permissible for a medical practitioner to give a patient suffering from a mortal disease a poisonous dose of opium or other narcotic drug in order to terminate his sufferings'.[270] He rejected this position as being contrary to the sacredness of human life, yet pointed to the distinction between giving opium with the intention to cause death and with the intention only to relieve pain while the drug might through its other effects hasten the fatal outcome of the disease. Saundby stopped short, however, of advocating such indirect euthanasia and concluded:

> It may be a choice of evils, but although the endeavour to alleviate pain is supported by general opinion, nothing should be done to warrant any suspicion that the sanctity of human life is trifled with by the medical profession.[271]

This position had been common among nineteenth-century physicians, who tended to share the view of many of their patients that the end of a person's life lay in God's hands and therefore must not be deliberately hastened. When doctors of that period spoke of 'euthanasia' or 'a good death', they usually meant dying under palliative care and pain relief, with moral and spiritual support. Influential here was the Evangelical belief that death had to be calmly

[270] Saundby, *Medical Ethics* (1907), p. 12.
[271] Ibid.

accepted rather than lamented. Moreover, according to Catholic doctrine, impending death should make the sick reflect upon Christ's suffering and sacrifice for humankind.[272] The question of voluntary active euthanasia and physician-assisted suicide had been raised, however, in Britain from the early 1870s, in articles for an educated public by the Birmingham schoolteacher Samuel D. Williams and the Oxford-educated philosopher Lionel Arthur Tollemache (1838–1919). They redefined 'euthanasia' as a morally justifiable act of mercy killing using high doses of opiates or chloroform. In their argumentation, the notion of the sanctity of life should be replaced with the concept of a 'worthwhile life'.[273]

For Tollemache, this meant that in an overcrowded population, from a Darwinian and utilitarian perspective, someone who was 'unhealthy, unhappy, and useless' should choose assisted suicide or 'modified *Harikari*', as he put it, in order to make room for someone 'happier, healthier, and more useful'.[274] As a precaution against abuse, Tollemache suggested that the 'concurrence of two or three medical men' might be required before 'granting the sick

---

[272] See Ian Dowbiggin, *A Concise History of Euthanasia: Life, Death, God, and Medicine* (Lanham, Rowan & Littlefield Publishers, 2005), pp. 39-46.

[273] Ibid., pp. 49-51; N. D. A. Kemp, *'Merciful release'. The history of the British euthanasia movement* (Manchester and New York, Manchester University Press, 2002), pp. 11-25.

[274] Lionel A. Tollemache, 'The Cure for Incurables' [annotated edition of essay first published in the *Fortnightly Review*, February 1873], in idem, *Stones of Stumbling* (London, Hodgson & Son, 1884), pp. 1-31, on pp. 4, 21.

man a release from his sufferings'.[275] Moreover he argued for the legalisation of physician-assisted suicide (as well as of suicide in general, which was then still a criminal offence), making it in this way subject to public scrutiny. Such legally sanctioned euthanasia performed by doctors would be less dangerous than tacitly accepting cases of hastening a patient's death 'by stealth' through the giving of narcotics.[276]

However, the ideas of Williams and Tollemache on this new form of euthanasia did not find acceptance in the British medical profession of the late nineteenth century. Characteristic was rather the pursuit of a 'good death' or euthanasia in its traditional sense, e.g. by William Munk (1816–1898), a Fellow of the Royal College of Physicians of London, who published in 1887 a monograph detailing techniques of palliative care of the dying. He advocated restricted administration of opium for pain relief and as a cardiac medicine, but warned against precipitating the patient's death by it.[277] Although, at the start of the twentieth century, medical officer of health for Willesden, London, C. E. Goddard, suggested in the context of Social Darwinist and eugenic thought mercy-killing in severe cases of terminal illness and of incurable mental deficiency, the official

---

[275] Ibid., p. 23.

[276] Ibid., pp. 27-28.

[277] Kemp, *'Merciful release'*, pp. 40-42; Dowbiggin, *History of Euthanasia*, pp. 44-46.

line of the British medical profession remained opposed to actively ending a patient's life. It would violate the Hippocratic Oath and be morally and legally unacceptable.[278] For example, when in 1904 the topic was raised again through newspaper reports on American discussions about euthanasia, an editorial of the *British Medical Journal* reminded its readers disapprovingly of Tollemache's article of over thirty years ago and made the professional stance once again clear:

> An unhappy sufferer who, worn out by pain and hopeless of relief, seeks to hasten the inevitable end, is probably scarcely to be held accountable for his action; in any case it is not for us to judge him. But a medical practitioner who should make himself the instrument of carrying out such a wish would be guilty of a crime against his patient, against society, and against his profession.[279]

Saundby's view on euthanasia was in line with this position. In sensitive issues such as euthanasia, as well as human experimentation and abortion, he paid careful attention to avoiding any conduct that might damage the reputation of the profession, even if patient interests might have justified a more liberal approach. His writing about medical ethics was not only about intra-professional mat-

---

[278] See Kemp, *'Merciful release'*, pp. 44-56.

[279] 'Euthanasia', *British Medical Journal*, June 11, 1904, pp. 1384-1386, on p. 1386.

ters, but also about advising colleagues to conduct themselves in a way that would support a public image of moral rectitude.

Conclusions

From the late eighteenth to the early twentieth century writings on medical ethics thus served various purposes. Preventing or mitigating conflict and competition between different groups in the medical profession was clearly one prominent aim. Until about the mid-nineteenth century this concerned mainly the professional relationships between physicians, surgeons and apothecaries; and after the creation of the General Medical Council in the late 1850s, predominantly the relations between licensed and unlicensed and between general and specialist (consulting) practitioners. Honourable, gentlemanly conduct was the ideal that authors of medical ethical works promoted. Such honourable professional conduct was always also seen as linked to moral behaviour in dealing with patients and in the relations with the public at large. Whether conceptualised as a sympathetic, compassionate attitude of a practitioner towards the ill, or as paternalistic consideration of their interests, the patient-oriented side of professional ethics was the other major theme of medico-ethical writing.

Ideally, professional and patient interests were seen as interacting harmoniously, except perhaps when patients sought the advice of multiple practitioners or wished to change their attending doctor. Writers on medical ethics therefore usually addressed readers beyond the profession, aiming to convince the public that their regularly trained medical attendant deserved their trust. At the same time, they tried to inculcate on fellow practitioners, and especially on incoming junior practitioners, a sense of intra-professional solidarity and of professional responsibility in their treatment of patients. However, in a number of areas nineteenth-century practitioners faced difficult moral choices, for example, in deciding between Caesarean section and destruction of the foetus in cases of severely obstructed labour. Other choices concerned the duty of confidentiality, such as the question of whether or not to disclose the venereal disease of a patient to a third person who was at risk of being infected; or, whether or not to inform the authorities about a case of illegal abortion in an attempt to stop a dangerous lay abortionist. Personal moral convictions as well as social, legal and professional norms came to bear on such situations. In the following two chapters, I will turn to these serious moral problems in nineteenth-century medicine.

Chapter 4

Craniotomy or Caesarean Section? An Ethical Issue in the Practice of Obstetrics

Introduction

One of the most dramatic conflicts in nineteenth-century medicine, literally involving life-or-death decisions, could occur in the practice of obstetrics. These were the rare but very serious cases of severely obstructed labour which were typically caused by the mother's pelvis being too narrow and deformed (usually because of rachitic disease), so that the baby could neither be delivered manually nor by use of the forceps. Practitioners had then the following alternatives: they could either perform a Caesarean section, which in the early decades of the nineteenth century ended with the woman's death in every third or even every second case, due to severe bleeding, inflammation and gangrene;[280] or they could perform the gruesome, ancient procedure of foetal craniotomy in which the unborn baby's skull was perforated with a sharp instrument, the brain substance destroyed and removed, and the skull reduced in size to make extraction with a hook or forceps possible. So, the tragic choice was between risking the life of the mother in the hope of delivering a living child; or sacrificing the unborn child's life in an attempt to save the mother. Even if the decision for craniotomy was made, maternal mortality was still between 20 and 40 per cent, in addition to the certain death of the foetus; and if a practitioner dared to perform a Caesarean section on the pregnant woman, the mortality for the baby was still around 30 per cent, besides the severe risks for the mother.[281] A third option, symphysiotomy, that is, cutting through the cartilage uniting the two pubic bones and widening the pelvis, was occasionally mentioned, but rarely

[280] Michael Ryan, 'Manual of Midwifery' (1841), partial reprint in Howard Brody, Zahra Meghani and Kimberley Greenwald (eds), *Michael Ryan's Writings on Medical Ethics* (Dordrecht, Springer, 2010), pp. 227-242, on pp. 237-238; Jacqueline H. Wolf, *Cesarean Section: An American History of Risk, Technology, and Consequence* (Baltimore, Johns Hopkins University Press, 2018), p. 22.

[281] Carl Capellmann, *Pastoral Medicine*, transl. by William Dassel (New York and Cincinnati, Fr. Pustet, 1879), pp. 18-19; Samuel C. Busey, 'Craniotomy Upon the Living Fetus is Not Justifiable', *American Journal of Obstetrics and Diseases of Women and Children* 17 (1884), pp. 176-193, on p. 178.

practised, as it could be insufficient and leave the woman with a painful disability.[282]

Christian and Secular Views among London Obstetricians

A source that reflects in detail on the dilemma is the *Manual of Midwifery* by the Irish-born physician Michael Ryan (see chapter 3, above), who practised in London between 1828, the year of the first edition of this manual, and 1840, the year of his death. In the following I refer to the posthumous fourth edition of his manual, which was published in 1841 and in part reprinted in 2010.[283]

In discussing the problem, Ryan made the intriguing observation that British doctors tended to decide for craniotomy of the foetus, whereas French, German and American

[282] Wolf, *Cesarean Section*, p. 32; James Blundell, *The Principles and Practice of Obstetricy, to which are added, Notes and Illustrations, by Thomas Castle* (Washington, Duff Green, 1834), pp. 362-363.

[283] Michael Ryan, 'Manual of Midwifery' (1841), partial reprint in Howard Brody, Zahra Meghani and Kimberley Greenwald (eds), *Michael Ryan's Writings on Medical Ethics* (Dordrecht, Springer, 2010), pp. 227-242. For Ryan's biography, see ibid., pp. 17-34; and for his wider views on medical ethics, see chapter 3, above.

obstetricians were more willing to perform a Caesarean section on the woman.[284] The moral justification of those British practitioners was, as Ryan noted, that 'the tree should be preferred to the fruit', or that the mother's life was more valuable than the life of the baby. The European and American preference for Caesarean section, Ryan thought, was motivated by the Christian belief – going back to Thomas Aquinas – that only a born, living baby could be baptised and thus be granted God's gift of an eternal afterlife, that is, it had to be born in order to be 'reborn'.[285]

Ryan disagreed to some extent with both positions. Referring to the Fifth Commandment, 'Thou shalt not kill', he firmly rejected the option of craniotomy on a living foetus. Only if the foetus had died in the womb would this procedure be permissible.[286] This matched the traditional role for the male practitioner to be called in by the midwife in order to remove a dead foetus.[287] Whether the foetus was still alive

---

[284] Ryan, 'Manual of Midwifery', p. 232. This statement appears to support Ornella Moscucci's claim that in the middle of the nineteenth century French, Catholic obstetricians were more ready to resort to Caesarean section than their British, Protestant colleagues. See her *The Science of Woman: Gynaecology and Gender in England, 1800-1929* (Cambridge, Cambridge University Press, 1993), pp. 141-143. It conflicts in part with Jacqueline Wolf's claim, *Cesarean Section*, pp. 36-37 and 43-44, that, for most of the nineteenth century, American doctors invariably chose craniotomy over Caesarean section.
[285] Ryan, 'Manual of Midwifery', p. 232.
[286] Ibid., p. 230.
[287] See Adrian Wilson, *Ritual and Conflict: The Social Relations of Childbirth in Early Modern England* (Farnham and Burlington, Ashgate, 2013), p. 224.

could, in Ryan's opinion, reliably be determined by listening for its heartbeats with the stethoscope (which had been introduced by French physician Renée Laennec in 1819) and a metroscope (i.e. an instrument for auscultating the uterus from the vagina).[288] However, he was also very reluctant to carry out the dangerous Caesarean operation on the living mother. Intrauterine baptism by applying the holy water with a syringe to the living foetus, or the membranes surrounding it, was in his view valid, citing a ruling of the theologians of the Sorbonne on this question from 1773.[289]

Ryan's advice was that the obstetrician should stand back and wait if vaginal delivery turned out to be impossible. In almost all cases the foetus would, compressed by the womb's contractions, perish before the woman, so that foetal craniotomy became then permissible.[290] Ryan's stance was in line with the Roman Catholic position, which had been clearly expressed in 1648 by the Sorbonne theologians in a reply to the medical faculty:

> [...] if the infant cannot be extracted without killing it, it cannot be extracted without committing a mortal sin, and that in such a case, it would be best to hold the

[288] Ryan, 'Manual of Midwifery', pp. 230-231.
[289] Ibid., p. 232.
[290] Ibid., p. 230.

maxim of St. Ambrose, – 'If one cannot be assisted without seriously injuring the other, it is best not to assist either.'[291]

Ryan also discussed the option of a Caesarean section, but concluded, in light of its high mortality, that it should be performed only if absolutely necessary.[292] He rejected as immoral and illegal the custom of previous centuries to give the decision between the mother's and infant's life to the husband respectively the child's father.[293] Ryan did not explicitly discuss the woman's will in this emergency situation, though in general obstetric practice he demanded that the woman or her close relatives be informed if an instrumental delivery, for example with the forceps, appeared to become necessary.[294]

He further discussed related issues, such as the question of whether the induction of premature labour was permissible if it was foreseeable that vaginal delivery would be impossible at the end of the pregnancy. His answer was, in line with the commandment not to kill, that such induction was allowed if the foetus had reached the stage of viability, which he put at seven and a half months' gestation.[295] He also considered cases where the woman had survived a Caesarean section and had become pregnant again. Should

---

[291] Ibid., p. 232.
[292] Ibid. p. 238.
[293] Ibid., pp. 231, 233.
[294] Ibid., p. 227.
[295] Ibid., pp. 228, 241.

therefore the Fallopian tubes be cut, to avoid a future pregnancy? His answer was 'no', as such interference in fertility was against Divine will. Ryan inveighed against Malthusian ideas on overpopulation, and polemically raised the question whether the husbands and other men shouldn't rather be castrated to prevent the need for Caesarean sections.[296]

Ryan wrote in part against a London colleague, James Blundell (1790–1878), professor of obstetrics at Guy's Hospital.[297] In his lectures, published in 1834 under the title *The Principles and Practice of Obstetricy,* Blundell discussed among others embryotomy and craniotomy. While he deemed embryotomy operations such as decapitation and dismemberment only to be necessary in the dead foetus, craniotomy on a still living foetus, though 'dreadful', as he emphasised, might sometimes be 'peremptorily' required for the safety of the mother.[298] As Blundell stated:

> By some, perhaps, it might be contended, that we are never justified in having recourse to craniotomy, unless the foetus be already dead, but this opinion is, I conceive erroneous. With the dogmas of the divine, it is not in my province to interfere, and I am glad of it; without, therefore, babbling about theology and syringes, I may be

[296] Ibid., pp. 229, 233-234, 239.

[297] For Blundell's biography, see J. H. Young, 'James Blundell (1790-1878): Experimental Physiologist and Obstetrician', *Medical History* 8 (1964), pp. 159-169.

[298] James Blundell, *The Principles and Practice of Obstetricy, to which are added, Notes and Illustrations, by Thomas Castle* (Washington, Duff Green, 1834), pp. 244-245, 330-331.

> permitted to remark, that in British obstetricy, the life, nay the preservation of the patient, from the graver lesions of the person, is to be looked upon as paramount to every consideration relating to the foetus; and when these require the sacrifice, craniotomy becomes justifiable.[299]

In order to clear the operation from being regarded as murder, Blundell was at pains to establish the medical indications that made craniotomy absolutely necessary, such as repeated failure of applying the forceps, with dangerous symptoms appearing in the mother, and severe contraction of her pelvis. He preferred, if possible, to craniotomise the already dead foetus, and so he provided signs of its death, including the coming off of the cuticle from the scalp, disruption of the skull's bones, and the stop of pulsations in the umbilical cord for 30 or 40 minutes.[300]

The Caesarean operation was, Blundell observed, 'sometimes' used in Britain and 'more frequently' on the Continent if delivery through the natural passages was impracticable. The method was apparently known since antiquity, named after Julius Caesar who was believed to have been delivered that way, but until the eighteenth century only as a procedure to be carried out after the woman had died, in

---

[299] Ibid., pp. 339-340.
[300] Ibid., pp. 340-344.

the hope of delivering a still living child.[301] At the time of Blundell's writing, Caesarean section on the living woman was a daring operation requiring, as he noted, a certain 'intrepidity' of the obstetrician, 'fortitude' of the woman, and a steady assistant with 'firm nerves' standing on either side of the bed to secure the woman if necessary.[302] This referred of course to the pre-anaesthetic era (inhalation anaesthesia being introduced only from the middle of the 1840s).

Blundell described the technique of the Caesarean operation in some detail, also drawing upon his experimental research on it in dogs and rabbits. Before closing the abdominal wound, he advised to cut the Fallopian tubes, and remove a small portion of them on both sides, in order to prevent a future pregnancy.[303] In the early 1830s Blundell was looking at reports of about 200 to 300 Caesarean sections performed on the European Continent over the previous decades, with a bit more than half of the women surviving the operation. On the British Isles, however, only two successful cases, i.e. cases in which the woman survived the section, were known then, one conducted by a surgeon, Mr Barlow of Blackburn, in 1793 and another by an Irish midwife, Mary Dunnally, who used a razor, in 1738.[304]

---

[301] See Alessandra Foscati, '"Nonnatus dictus quod caeso defunctae matris utero prodiit". Postmortem Caesarean Section in the Late Middle Ages and Early Modern Period', *Social History of Medicine* 32 (2019), pp. 465-480.
[302] Blundell, *Principles and Practice of Obstetricy*, p. 349.
[303] Ibid., pp. 349-352.
[304] Ibid., pp. 352-357.

Blundell acknowledged that the hope for baptism of the living child might have induced some women to submit to Caesarean section, but fully aware of the risks, he held against this what he called the 'British Rule of Obstetricy': not to remove the foetus by Caesarean incisions if it could be extracted through the natural passages. The implication of this rule was that craniotomy and vaginal extraction of the dead foetus was preferable to the risky Caesarean operation. Blundell did, however, accept the case for relatively early Caesarean section, i.e. before the woman had become exhausted, if her 'cordial assent' to the operation had been obtained.[305] This emphasis on consent matched the practice of other nineteenth-century doctors who, as Jacqueline Wolf has pointed out in her recent history of Caesarean section in America, 'did not perform an operation without the consensus of everyone present', including the woman herself and her friends.[306]

Finally, Blundell considered options for preventing the necessity of Caesarean sections in women known to have a too narrow pelvis. Abstinence from sexual intercourse was one suggestion, but, admitting that this may be difficult to achieve in marriage, he proposed, as mentioned, section of the Fallopian tubes to induce sterility. If pregnancy had occurred, he suggested in the early stages abortive medicines

---

[305] Ibid., pp. 353-354.

[306] Wolf, *Cesarean Section*, p. 23. This typically referred, however, to white patients only. Ibid., p. 24.

or instrumental destruction of the 'ovum', i.e. the early embryo, by passing a sound through the mouth of the uterus or driving a trocar through its walls.[307] These were just suggestions, to be sure, but they provoked severe criticism by Ryan who considered them to be immoral interventions into Divine will and pointed out that in English law abortion was a felony.[308] For the end of the pregnancy, Blundell weighed up craniotomy versus Caesarean section, and in line with the 'British Rule of Obstetricy' he came to the following conclusion:

> Observe, it is a rule – an axiom in British midwifery, that we are never to deliver by the Caesarian operation, provided we may, in any way, deliver by the natural passages. [...] if [...] we were once to establish the principle, that the Caesarian delivery may be used as a substitute for delivery by the perforator, there would, I fear, be too many cases in which it would be needlessly adopted, and men would now and then, not to say frequently, perform this operation under circumstances in which it ought never to have been dreamed of. Where, therefore, the embryotomic delivery is practicable, let this be preferred.[309]

In contrast to Ryan, Blundell thus addressed the problem of severely obstructed labour by permitting craniotomy on

[307] Blundell, *Principles and Practice of Obstetricy*, pp. 360-361.
[308] Ryan, 'Manual of Midwifery', pp. 240-241.
[309] Blundell, *Principles and Practice of Obstetricy*, p. 361.

the still living foetus as well as by proposing preventative methods including sterilization and, what we would now call, therapeutic abortions. Blundell's position may be called a secular one, in which medical considerations were paramount. It clearly differed from Ryan's Christian, specifically Roman Catholic views on the problem, which prohibited these measures.

Blundell's secular position on the permissibility of craniotomy, even if the foetus was still alive, was shared in the early 1840s by his colleague Francis Henry Rambotham (1801–1868), a consultant and lecturer in obstetrics and forensic medicine at the London Hospital, in his textbook on obstetric medicine and surgery. Although Rambotham was sympathetic to the view of those who argued that human life was solely dependent on God's will and that therefore the living foetus must not be destroyed by human hand, he felt that such objections were only valid if craniotomy was performed without serious consideration. In his opinion, however, there were 'strong and numerous' arguments to prefer the life of the mother over the life of the unborn child if the situation required to make a decision for one or the other. He also regarded foetal craniotomy as justified if the woman was not in immediate danger, in order to spare her severe injuries that would cause her to suffer for the rest of her life.[310] Rambotham was explicit about his reasons for this preference:

[...] I may remark that the mother is bound to the world by many social, moral, and religious ties; she has shared the enjoyments, as well as the cares of life; she has her feelings and affections, her fears and hopes; she is dependent on others, and other are dependent on her; when she dies, there is left a blank, which, to some surviving, never can be filled. Not so, however, with the unborn infant. Although, in dying, some personal pain may be experienced, yet the agony of mind it cannot suffer: it has no affections, no dependents; its existence centres almost exclusively in itself; – except to its nearest relatives, then, its death, cannot be greatly felt. And, notwithstanding we cannot estimate life relatively, as we can any other possession [...] yet we are surely justified, in a political, if not in a moral point of view, in preferring the preservation of the strong to the weak, the healthy to the diseased, and the mother of a family to the unborn foetus, provided one or the other must in all probability be sacrificed. From these considerations, we prefer, whenever we have a choice, the mother's safety to the infant's life [...].[311]

---

[310] Francis H. Rambotham, *The Principles and Practice of Obstetric Medicine and Surgery, in Reference to the Process of Parturition.* A New Edition, from the Enlarged and Revised London Edition (Philadelphia, Lea & Blanchard, 1845), pp. 208-209.

[311] Ibid., p. 209.

Rambotham thus argued for preferring the mother in light of her status as a person and because of her social importance. These considerations were for him more compelling than religious objections to sacrificing the unborn foetus, which would neither experience the same kind of suffering as an adult nor be missed in the way a mother would be. Rambotham noted that this was the usual position held in British midwifery, whereas French, German, Italian and some American obstetricians regarded craniotomy only as permissible after the foetus had died.[312] He furthermore considered Caesarean section as a possible alternative to foetal craniotomy, recognising that the former might be necessary in cases of severe distortion of the mother's pelvis or obstruction of the birth canal by a tumour. However, as he pointed out regarding the Caesarean operation, 'in Britain we never substitute it for craniotomy by choice, but only have recourse to it when no other mode of delivery is practicable.'[313] Rambotham made this statement in the context of his observation that the mother had survived in only three cases of Caesarean section out of less than thirty by then attempted in the British Isles.[314] He acknowledged that in Europe, especially in Catholic countries, Caesarean section had been performed more frequently and with more success, as the decision for it tended

[312] Ibid., p. 209, footnote.
[313] Ibid., p. 221.
[314] Ibid., pp. 145-146, 221.

to be made there earlier in cases of obstructed labour when the woman had still sufficient strength to withstand the operation. Rambotham also assumed that women in those countries were more influenced by the clergy than in Britain and agreed more readily to a Caesarean section out of a sense of religious duty, in the hope that a living child would be delivered and baptised, thus giving it 'the benefit of admission within the pale of the Christian church'.[315]

Moving away from Craniotomy, towards Caesarean Section

With the introduction of anaesthesia with ether and chloroform in 1846 and 1847 respectively, of Lister's antisepsis from the late 1860s, and technical improvements such as suturing the cut uterus from the 1880s, the argument started to turn in favour of the Caesarean section and against craniotomy.[316] An early British opponent of craniotomy was William Tyler Smith (1815–1873), an obstetric physician and lecturer in midwifery and women's diseases at St. Mary's Hospital, London. As Smith reported to the Obstetrical Society of London in 1859, in British practice craniotomy was performed in about 1 in every 340 labours, which amounted for England and Wales to about 1,800 foetal deaths per year. In most cases, he assumed, the foetus was still alive when

---

[315] Ibid., p. 146.
[316] Busey, 'Craniotomy'; Wolf, *Cesarean Section*, pp. 44-46.

the decision for craniotomy was made. In addition, maternal mortality for the procedure was, according to his figures, about 1 in 5, which meant that, again in England and Wales, over 350 pregnant women died annually in connection with craniotomy. Accordingly, Smith aimed at the abolition of the procedure from obstetric practice whenever the foetus was alive and viable.[317] In cases of moderate deformity of the mother's pelvis he advocated induction of premature labour around the seventh month of gestation, which would significantly reduce the risk for the woman and give the child a fair chance of survival. He furthermore believed that most British obstetricians would recognise the propriety, in cases of severe pelvic distortion, to induce labour in the early or middle months of pregnancy, i.e. to produce a miscarriage in the interest of saving the woman.[318] In many other situations, he claimed, where craniotomy had been performed, this could have been avoided by turning of the foetus and skilful use of the forceps.[319] As Smith emphasised, anaesthesia with chloroform enabled a much wider application of the forceps than had been possible in the past.[320] In this way also the Caesarean operation, which Smith thought to be 'full of danger' and only slightly less

---

[317] W. Tyler Smith, 'On the Abolition of Craniotomy from Obstetric Practice, in All Cases Where the Foetus is Living and Viable', *Transactions of the Obstetrical Society of London* 1 (1859), pp. 21-50, on pp. 21-23.

[318] Ibid., p. 26.

[319] Ibid., pp. 26-30.

[320] Ibid., p. 39.

deadly for the mother than craniotomy for the child, might be avoided.[321]

From about the middle of the nineteenth century the issue of Caesarean section versus craniotomy became a common topic of Catholic writing on ethical questions of medical practice.[322] For example, the German Catholic physician Carl Capellmann (1841–1898), who practised in Aix-la-Chapelle, addressed the issue in the 1870s in his work *Pastoral Medicine* within a chapter on the implications of the Fifth Commandment.[323] He deplored that in his day craniotomy on the living foetus was being seen as justified when the woman was unwilling to consent to a Caesarean section; and he fiercely added:

> Is perforation of the living foetus allowed as a means of saving the mother? Certainly not, because it is a direct killing of the foetus, which is always forbidden.[324]

---

[321] Ibid., pp. 22, 28.

[322] For detailed discussions of Catholic positions in the nineteenth-century debate on Caesarean section versus craniotomy, see Joseph G. Ryan, 'The Chapel and the Operating Room: The Struggle of Roman Catholic Clergy, Physicians, and Believers with the Dilemmas of Obstetric Surgery, 1800-1900', *Bulletin of the History of Medicine* 76 (2002), pp. 461-494; Jolien Gijbels, 'L'omniprésence de la religion. Les médecins belges et le dilemme obstetrical (1840-1880)', *Annales de démographie historique* 138/1 (2020), pp. 207-235.

[323] Capellmann, *Pastoral Medicine*, pp. 17-20. For a discussion of Capellmann's book, see David F. Kelly, *The Emergence of Catholic Medical Ethics in North America: An Historical-Methodological-Bibliographical Study* (New York and Toronto, Edwin Mellen Press, 1979), pp. 70-74.

[324] Capellmann, *Pastoral Medicine*, p. 17.

Analysing published reports on Caesarean sections between 1750 and 1861, he tried to demonstrate that the operation had become 'comparatively safe', with 54 out of 100 mothers surviving it and about 70 per cent of the children delivered this way being saved. This he compared with data on craniotomy, in which nearly 40 per cent of the mothers had died, in addition to the certain death of the child.[325] Capellmann therefore made the argument that the pregnant woman should agree to a Caesarean section to save the child's life.[326] In practice, though, he recommended that if the woman's consent to the operation could not be obtained, the obstetrician should await the death of either mother or child and then assist the surviving one, i.e. taking the Catholic approach to the situation.[327]

In the late nineteenth century craniotomy began to be seen as outdated, and was even suspected to be misused as a form of late abortion. As American Protestant physician Samuel C. Busey put it in 1883 in his presidential address to the Washington Obstetrical and Gynecological Society:

> Craniotomy offers no hope […], but proclaims from the altar of professional justification death by violence to the fetuses of women who are physically incapacitated to give birth to a living child. Nay, more, it offers immunity

[325] Ibid., pp. 18-19.
[326] Ibid., pp. 23-24.
[327] Ibid., p. 20.

> from the travail of labor, and protection from the annoyances of maternity to those who have accepted the pleasures of concubinage or wedlock, and have become copartners in the creation of a new being and a new soul to live forever, but who cannot complete the highest and noblest purpose of woman's creation. So repulsive does it present itself in this aspect, that many who have advocated and performed it recoil from its repetition upon the same woman.[328]

From the medical point of view, the decision against craniotomy and for Caesarean section (or a related procedure such as the operative removal of the uterus) was increasingly influenced by measurements taken of the pregnant woman's pelvis ('pelvimetry'). As Busey summarized, professional opinion appeared to consolidate on the view that craniotomy was inadmissible if the conjugate diameter (between the lower margin of the symphysis and the sacro-coccygeal joint) was less than two and a half inches; only if it was greater, craniotomy might be safer for the mother than a Caesarean section.[329] Reviewing the recent medical literature on the question, Busey came down firmly on the side of Caesarean section, concluding that it was better to 'offer chances to two lives rather than take one which cannot assure the safety of the other'.[330] More generally, in the late

[328] Busey, 'Craniotomy', p. 180.
[329] Ibid., pp. 182-183.
[330] Ibid., p. 193.

nineteenth and early twentieth centuries decisions to perform a Caesarean section, as opposed to attempting vaginal delivery, often relied on the results of pelvic measurements.[331]

Yet, the ethical issue of craniotomy on the living foetus versus Caesarean operation on the pregnant woman was still a topic in medical as well as religious fora. In March 1884, the Vatican issued a prohibition of teaching craniotomy in Catholic schools, and in August 1889 it endorsed its opposition to craniotomy and any operations that would directly kill the foetus or the pregnant mother.[332] In 1893, ten years after Busey's speech in Washington DC, the Sunderland surgeon James Murphy included the matter in his opening address to the Section of Obstetric Medicine and Gynaecology at the British Medical Association's annual meeting in Newcastle upon Tyne. In his view, craniotomy of the living foetus was no longer justifiable, as the risk of the mother's death after Caesarean section had gone down to 10 per cent or less. He urged in particular the older generation of practitioners, who would not visit the operating theatres, to recognise this and to find in appropriate cases a

---

[331] Wolf, *Cesarean Section*, pp. 54-59. See also Mark William Skippen, *Obstetric practice and cephalopelvic disproportion in Glasgow between 1840 and 1900* (PhD thesis, University of Glasgow, 2009).

[332] Ryan, 'The Chapel and the Operating Room', pp. 480, 483; Julia Fleming, 'The Ethics of Therapeutic Abortion and an American Catholic Medical School: Charles Coppens, S.J. and the Creighton Medical College', *Journal of Religion & Society*, Supplement Series, Supplement 7 (2011), pp. 112-133, on pp. 115-117.

neighbouring colleague who was able to perform the Caesarean operation. Murphy also thought that the objection that the woman would not consent to Caesarean section was no longer valid, because 'a successful operating surgeon' was 'capable of getting the patient's consent when an operation is necessary'.[333]

In the same year, 1893, the topic featured with two articles in the *American Ecclesiastical Review*, a journal for the Catholic clergy. In the first contribution, Philadelphia physician M. O'Hara advocated Caesarean section over craniotomy, citing Murphy in support of his position. O'Hara predicted that those 'few' who still believed in the 'warrantable destruction of the foetus' would 'go to the wall' and that, in line with Catholic teaching, craniotomy should be seen as 'a violation of moral law and a crime against society'.[334] In the other article, William H. Parish, a professor in the Woman's Medical College of Philadelphia and a non-Catholic, took a more moderate position, acknowledging that the life of the woman had to be preferred over the life of the foetus, if the situation required the choice. However, he pointed out that craniotomy had become a rare procedure now that Caesarean section could be performed with much greater safety for

---

[333] James Murphy, 'An Address Delivered at the Opening of the Section of Obstetric Medicine and Gynaecology. At the Annual Meeting of the British Medical Association held in Newcastle-upon-Tyne, August, 1893', *British Medical Journal*, August 26, 1893, pp. 453-455, on p. 454. On the problems of consent, see chapter 2, above.

[334] M. O'Hara, 'Caesarean Section versus Craniotomy', *American Ecclesiastical Review* 9 (1893), pp. 360-363.

the woman. Parish supported Caesarean section, which would not carry much higher risk to the mother than perforation and extraction of the foetus. If performed under favourable conditions, about 95 per cent of the mothers would recover from either procedure.[335] In July 1895, the Vatican issued a ruling against medical abortion.[336] Subsequently, drawing upon the medical opinions of Parish, O'Hara and Murphy, the Belgian-American Jesuit priest Charles Coppens (1835–1920), who taught medical jurisprudence at the Catholic Creighton Medical College in Omaha, Nebraska, argued in his 1897 textbook on moral principles in medical practice against craniotomy as the killing of an innocent human being. In particular, he rejected the argument that it might be justifiable as a form of self-defence of the mother.[337]

Conclusions

Towards the end of the nineteenth century, then, the debate over craniotomy versus Caesarean section had shifted in favour of the latter. This was largely due to developments in

---

[335] W. H. Parish, 'The Present State of Craniotomy in the Medical Profession', *American Ecclesiastical Review* 9 (1893), pp. 363-366.

[336] Ryan, 'The Chapel and the Operating Room', pp. 491-492.

[337] Charles Coppens, *Moral Principles and Medical Practice: The Basis of Medical Jurisprudence* (New York, Cincinnati and Chicago, Benziger Brothers, 1897), pp. 50-54. For discussions of Coppens' book, see Kelly, *Emergence of Catholic Medical Ethics*, pp. 110-117; Fleming, 'The Ethics of Therapeutic Abortion', pp. 123-127.

surgery that made the Caesarean operation much safer than it had been in the early and middle decades of the century. However, the Catholic position, which denounced the killing of the foetus as violating the Fifth Commandment, also played a role in this development, providing a moral reason to pursue the option of a Caesarean section, even when the risks to the woman were very substantial, as they were during most of the nineteenth century. In making the decision between Caesarean section and craniotomy, medical assessment of the expected best outcome for the mother played the key role, but religious views could exclude the option of craniotomy on the living foetus and favour, despite its high risk, the Caesarean operation, which might result in a living baby that could be baptised. To prevent the emergency situation from arising, induction of premature labour was regarded as acceptable in women who were known to have a too narrow pelvis (having experienced the problem in a previous birth). Such induction was meant to be carried out preferably when the foetus had become viable in about the seventh month, so that the lives of both mother and child might be saved. In cases of severe deformation of the mother's pelvis, some obstetricians were prepared to induce a miscarriage already in the early or middle months of pregnancy in order to save the woman. Yet, abortion was classed in nineteenth-century Britain, as well as in America and European countries, as a crime, so authors addressing the topic of induction were keen to emphasize that this latter procedure had to be viewed differently from illegal abortions.[338]

---

[338] See e.g. Busey, 'Craniotomy', pp. 184-185; Robert Saundby, *Medical Ethics: A Guide to Professional Conduct*, 2nd edn (London, Charles Griffin & Company, 1907), pp. 64, 123.

Chapter 5

Should a Doctor Tell? Conflicts over Confidentiality in Abortion and Venereal Diseases

Introduction[339]

Throughout the nineteenth century, English statutory law included severe penalties for abortions. They had first been made a statutory offence with Lord Ellenborough's Act of 1803, which punished the perpetrator with death if the woman had been 'quick with child' (i.e. after the first foetal movements were felt by the pregnant woman in the fourth or fifth month). Pre-quickening abortions were punishable with a variety of lesser penalties. While the Offences Against the Person Act of 1837 abolished the death penalty for abortions after quickening, it also gave up the distinction between pre-quickening and post-quickening, making any artificial termination of pregnancy a felony which could be

[339] This chapter draws upon my discussion of the topic in Andreas-Holger Maehle, *Contesting Medical Confidentiality: Origins of the Debate in the United States, Britain, and Germany* (Chicago and London, University of Chicago Press, 2016).

punished with transportation for no less than fifteen years or imprisonment for up to three years. Abortion then was no longer a capital offence. Yet, if the woman died from the intervention, the abortionist could still face the death penalty for murder. With the Offences Against the Person Act of 1861, abortion could carry a maximum penalty of lifelong imprisonment. Importantly, the offence was explicitly made punishable even if the pregnant woman had induced an abortion on herself, without the help of another person.[340]

However, the severity of the punishment contrasted with nineteenth-century public opinion, in which early abortions before quickening were widely deemed acceptable. It also contrasted with legal reality, in which relatively few cases actually came to trial, while abortion was frequently used to limit family size. Those cases that did come to the attention of the authorities where typically abortions performed by lay practitioners using instruments that had led to injury and severe infection (blood poisoning) in the woman.[341]

Regular medical practitioners could hide performing an abortion behind claims of necessary treatment, but risked being erased from the Register of the General Medical

---

[340] John Keown, *Abortion, doctors and the law: Some aspects of the legal regulation of abortion in England from 1803 to 1982* (Cambridge, Cambridge University Press, 2002), pp. 26-27.

[341] Barbara Brookes, *Abortion in England, 1900-1967* (London, Croom Helm, 1988), pp. 22-23.

Council if it came to light that they had carried out an 'illegal operation'. Indeed, the Minutes of the GMC regularly recorded cases of medical practitioners being struck off for this reason.[342] Many doctors would avoid this risk by refusing to perform terminations of pregnancy in the first place, but a difficult situation could still arise for them if they were called to attend to a woman who was experiencing serious complications from an illegal abortion. Should they then report the case to the police or public prosecutor, in an attempt to identify and help bringing to justice a dangerous abortionist, or should they adhere to their professional duty of confidentiality and thus protect their patient from possible prosecution? This dilemma became a topic of controversial discussions among lawyers and medical professionals in the late nineteenth and early twentieth centuries, triggered by two significant legal cases, *Kitson v. Playfair* (1896) and *R v. Annie Hodgkiss* (1914). In the first half of this chapter I discuss this issue of disclosure in abortion cases, and then, in the second half, turn to another set of problems of medical confidentiality, the warning of contacts of patients with a venereal disease and the disclosure of VD infection in divorce trials.

---

[342] Russell G. Smith, *Medical Discipline: The Professional Conduct Jurisdiction of the General Medical Council, 1858-1990* (Oxford, Clarendon Press, 1994), p. 105. On the disciplinary role of the GMC, see chapter 1 above in the present volume.

The *Kitson v. Playfair* Trial and its Implications for Medical Confidentiality

Remarkably, the *Kitson v. Playfair* trial, in March 1896, initially was not about abortion, but a libel case, in which Mrs Linda Kitson accused her brother-in-law, the London obstetrician and gynaecologist William Smoult Playfair (1836–1903) of having disclosed a miscarriage of hers to her absent husband's family, as it seemed to prove her adultery. Because of persistent gynaecological problems, Linda Kitson had been examined by Playfair jointly with her usual doctor, Muzio Williams, in February 1894. On detecting remnants of placenta in her womb, Playfair concluded that she must have had a recent miscarriage – a shocking finding for him, as he knew that she had been away from her husband, Arthur Kitson, for well over a year. Arthur had stayed behind in Australia for business reasons, when Linda had left for England together with their two daughters in late 1892. While Playfair was aware that Linda Kitson had had a miscarriage shortly before her departure from Australia, he suspected adultery, and put before her the alternative to either leave London, thus breaking off all relations with his family, or to give him assurances that her husband had secretly visited England in the last three months. Otherwise, family honour would demand that he informed his wife, Arthur Kitson's sister. With Linda being evasive about a recent visit of her husband and unwilling to leave, Playfair told his wife, and subsequently, at her instigation, her older brother, Sir James Kitson. The latter had paid Linda Kitson and her daughters an annual allowance of £400 while her husband was abroad. On hearing the 'news' about her apparent adultery, Sir James stopped the payments. Linda subsequently sued Playfair and his wife for slander and libel. Playfair was found guilty, and Linda Kitson was awarded the then very high sum of £12,000 in damages. Upon appeal, an out of court settlement between the parties agreed on the reduced sum of £9,200.[343]

The verdict against Playfair had much to do with class and gender related perceptions, in which Linda Kitson gained sympathy with the jury as a middle-class lady who had been accused of immoral behaviour and pressurised by her medical brother-in-law, who failed to act as a gentleman towards her. The trial raised, however, more general questions about the limits of medical confidentiality, and specifically about disclosure of abortions (although no suggestion had been made that a criminal abortion had been performed in Linda's case). The issue of abortion and confidentiality was brought up during the trial by the judge, Sir Henry Hawkins (1817–1907), by way of a comparison.

As part of the trial, expert witnesses were heard in order to establish the professional conventions regarding medical

---

[343] Angus McLaren, 'Privileged Communications: Medical Confidentiality in Late Victorian Britain', *Medical History 37* (1993), pp. 129-147. See also Maehle, *Contesting Medical Confidentiality*, pp. 74-75.

confidentiality. One of them, Sir John Williams, like Playfair a prominent obstetrician, named three situations in which it was thought justifiable for a medical practitioner to disclose confidential patient information: if the medical evidence was required in a court of law; in order to inform the public prosecutor of an intended or committed crime; and to protect the practitioner's wife and children. Sir William Broadbent, a senior fellow of the Royal College of Physicians (RCP) in London, confirmed Williams' assessment, but was somewhat hesitant about the third scenario (which Playfair might have used as an excuse for his breach of confidentiality by claiming to protect the interests of his wife's family).[344] When Williams, during cross examination, stated that it was up to the medical practitioner to decide when to disclose confidential information, Justice Hawkins intervened, putting a hypothetical case to him:

> Suppose a medical man were called in to attend a woman, and in the course of his professional attendance he discovers that she has attempted to procure an abortion. That being a crime under the law, would it be his duty to go and tell the Public Prosecutor?[345]

Williams responded by claiming that the Royal College of Physicians had answered this very question with 'yes', upon which Hawkins replied: 'Then all I can say is that it

[344] Cf. Maehle, *Contesting Medical Confidentiality*, p. 76.
[345] 'Kitson v. Playfair and Wife', *The Times*, March 26, 1896.

will make me very chary in the selection of my medical man.'[346] Furthermore, in his summing-up statement at the end of the trial, Hawkins returned to his example of a woman requiring medical help after an attempted abortion. It would be 'a monstrous cruelty', he said, if the doctor then reported her to the public prosecutor or the police.[347]

These remarks by a High Court judge, apparently condoning not to report an illegal abortion in order to protect the woman concerned, received considerable attention in the medical press. The editors of the *Lancet* commented that confidentiality might only be breached for 'overpowering reasons' and that a medical practitioner should have weighty information to support the allegation of a crime such as abortion before reporting the case to the authorities.[348] When an anonymous 'young practitioner' asked in a letter to the editors whether he should report to the police a young, unmarried woman who had confessed to him an illegal abortion attempt but was now recovering, their answer was 'no', they did not think that it was a medical man's duty to inform the authorities under such circumstances.[349] A legal correspondent to the *British Medical Journal* endorsed Hawkins' view. It was legally correct, he argued, because the secret was the patient's, not the doctor's, and the

[346] Ibid.
[347] 'Kitson v. Playfair and Wife', *The Times*, March 28, 1896; 'Kitson v. Playfair and Wife', *British Medical Journal* 1896, p. 883.
[348] 'Kitson v. Playfair', *The Lancet* 147 (1896), pp. 1292-1293.
[349] 'Professional Confidences', ibid., p. 1524.

woman's confidence rested on the implied understanding that her doctor would use the information about the abortion in her interest only. If, however, the abortion was merely *planned* to be carried out, the doctor would need to inform the authorities about this – otherwise he might make himself an accessory to the crime.[350] Another correspondent, signing M.D., advised caution, as Hawkins' words had only the status of *obiter dictum*, that is, of an opinion from the bench that was not binding for other judges, and could therefore not be taken as a guide for doctors' conduct.[351]

In late 1895, a few months before the *Kitson v. Playfair* case came to court, the Royal College of Physicians had already decided to form a committee and to seek legal advice on the question of what doctors should do if they were confronted with a case in which an illegal abortion was admitted to them, or where they suspected that one had taken place. Sir John Williams and Sir William Broadbent were both members of this committee. By the end of April 1896, they had obtained advice from the lawyers Edward Clarke QC (1841–1931), a former solicitor general, and Horace Avory (1851–1935). Clarke and Avory assured the RCP that it was not against the law if a doctor performed an abortion,

---

[350] 'The Obligation of Professional Secrecy. Medical and Legal Opinions I. – The Legal Issues. [By a Legal Correspondent.]', *British Medical Journal* 1896, April 4, pp. 869-870.

[351] M. D., 'Professional Secrecy and the Law', ibid., pp. 871-872.

or even destroyed a foetus during labour, if this was necessary to save the woman's life. If a medical practitioner believed, or got to know, that a *criminal* abortion had been performed on the woman he was treating, he should provide medical care for her to the best of his skill. This would *not* turn him into an accessory after the fact (as long as he did not do anything to help the woman escaping justice); and not reporting a merely suspected illegal abortion would not amount to concealment of a crime. If the doctor learned about a planned abortion, and obtained the abortionist's name, he should warn the latter that he had been informed (presumably with the intention to deter the abortionist from carrying out the procedure). Clarke and Avory concluded in general terms that it was left to the medical practitioner's discretion whether to report or not to report a particular case to the authorities and what to do if a pregnancy endangered a woman's life.[352]

Against the wishes of the RCP, its committee report was subsequently published in the journals *The Scalpel* and *Medical Press*,[353] and Robert Saundby referred to Clarke and Avory's advice in his guidebook *Medical Ethics* in 1907. Somewhat overstating their advice, Saundby claimed that it was 'to the effect that a medical man should not reveal facts

[352] A. M. Cooke, *A History of the Royal College of Physicians of London*, vol. 3 (Oxford, Clarendon Press, 1972), pp. 980-981.
[353] Ibid., p. 981.

which had come to his knowledge in the course of his professional duties, even in so extreme a case where there were grounds to suspect that a criminal offence had been committed'.[354]

In spite of such guidance, the question of whether medical practitioners should report illegal abortions remained controversial. In 1912, for example, in a case near Liverpool, where a woman had died from peritonitis after an illegal abortion, a police superintendent criticised during the coroner's inquest the deceased patient's doctor for not having reported the case before her death, so that the name of the abortionist might have been obtained from her. The doctor, however, defended himself saying that he had been bound to confidentiality and that he had the duty to do the best for his patient. The coroner agreed with him.[355] And a year later, the RCP received from the Local Government Board a query whether doctors of public hospitals were obliged to report cases where they suspected that a criminal abortion had been performed, or whether they had to protect patient confidentiality. The RCP responded by sending a copy of Clarke and Avory's legal advice of 1896.[356]

---

354 Saundby, *Medical Ethics*, pp. 113-114.

355 'Professional Secrecy', *The Lancet* 181 (1913), p. 52.

356 Cooke, *History of the Royal College*, vol. 3, pp. 981-982.

The Annie Hodgkiss Case and Disclosure of Illegal Abortion

Soon after, in 1914/15, the issue flared up again through another legal case. In December 1914, at the Birmingham Assizes, Annie Hodgkiss stood accused of having caused the death of a thirty-two-year-old single woman, Ellen Agnes Armstrong, by having performed an illegal abortion on her. From witness statements taken as part of the coroner's inquest, one can reconstruct Armstrong's tragic story.[357]

In early September 1914, then being about four or five months pregnant, Ellen Armstrong went to see an abortionist in Birmingham. The man who had gotten her pregnant, Bert Annise, was ignoring her, and, as she later told her father and her aunt, she would 'rather die than have the disgrace' and go on with the pregnancy. Her house doctor, Arthur William Aldridge, had in vain tried to persuade her to continue the pregnancy by offering to write a sick note over full six months for the company that employed her. The abortionist apparently used a sharp instrument and subsequently placed a rubber tube into her womb to keep the mouth of the uterus open. Later on the day of the procedure, Ellen went to see her aunt, Roseanna Oughton, initially saying she would like to stay at her house for a few days as her employer was short of work, but then confessing that she

---

[357] R v. Annie Hodgkiss: Coroner's Depositions, ASSI 13/44, Box 2, Birmingham Autumn Assizes 1914, fol. 1-17, National Archives, Kew.

had a pregnancy terminated. She refused to tell her aunt who the woman was who had performed the 'operation'. When her father visited her later on, she did not give him the name but only an address (which was different from that of Annie Hodgkiss). On 19 September, about two weeks after the procedure, a medical practitioner, Francis Joseph Johnson Orton, was called to Mrs Oughton's house, as Ellen was having a miscarriage, giving birth to an about five-month-old dead foetus. About a week later her temperature was rising, as Orton noted, and upon his questioning, she admitted that 'something had been done' to bring about the miscarriage. As Ellen's condition deteriorated with her temperature rising further and vomiting setting in, her father called for Dr Aldridge, who saw her on 29 September and arranged her admission to Birmingham's Women's Hospital at Sparkhill. The surgeon in charge of her case there, John Farmeaux Jordan, diagnosed acute inflammation and an abscess of the womb on the 30th and operated the following day. However, Ellen developed a general infection and blood poisoning, and died in the hospital on 16 October. The post-mortem examination on the following day, which Aldridge attended, confirmed a puncture wound, presumably caused by a sharp instrument, at the top of the vagina, an injury which Jordan had already seen during the operation. Moreover, the post-mortem showed septic endometritis and signs of generalised infection with abscesses in the lungs.

While Ellen Armstrong was in hospital, Dr Aldridge had visited her twice, and on the second occasion, on 11 October, she had admitted that an 'operation' had been carried out on her, and had given him the name and address of the person who had done it. However, Aldridge had not informed the police about the illegal abortion, nor had Orton, who had, however, told the surgeon, Mr Jordan, about it. Eventually, Jordan did report the case to the police after the post-mortem. Two police officers went to see Mrs Hodgkiss on 19 October and charged her with having caused Ellen Armstrong's death by performing an 'illegal operation' on her to procure an abortion. The police search of Hodgkiss's house produced some knitting pins and a 'crotchet', an instrument with small steel hooks. Among the belongings of Ellen at her aunt's house, the police found a letter with postmark 4 September containing a note by Hodgkiss confirming a meeting on Saturday morning (5 September). However, while Hodgkiss admitted that the note had been written by her, she denied having written Armstrong's address on the envelope. The police suspected that Ellen Armstrong had sent a self-addressed envelope to Hodgkiss, which was then used to post the note about the date of the appointment.

This letter was the only written piece of evidence linking Ellen Armstrong to the suspected abortionist, Annie Hodgkiss.

Horace Avory, who had meanwhile been appointed as a judge and was presiding over Annie Hodgkiss's trial, was deeply disappointed that no formal statement usable in court had been obtained from Ellen Armstrong before she died. In his address to the grand jury, on 1 December 1914, he expressed his frustration, as this meant that there was no justification for finding Hodgkiss guilty of murder. As Avory stated:

> I can see no evidence, as the case now stands, which will justify you in finding a true bill against the prisoner for murder. The law provides that in the case of any person who is seriously ill, and who, in the opinion of a medical man, is not likely to recover, the evidence of such a person may be taken by a Justice of the Peace. Under circumstances like those in the present case, I cannot doubt that it is the duty of the medical man to communicate with the Police, or with the Authorities, in order that one or other of those steps may be taken for the purpose of the administration of justice. [...] It may be the moral duty of the medical man, even in cases where the patient is not dying, or not unlikely to recover, to communicate with the Authorities when he sees good reason to believe that a criminal offence has been committed. However that may be, I cannot doubt that in such a case as

the present, where the woman was, in the opinion of the medical man, likely to die, and therefore her evidence was likely to be lost, it was his duty, and that some one of those gentlemen ought to have done it in this case.[358]

In essence, Avory reprimanded the doctors involved in Armstrong's care for having failed to report her case to the police before her death and blamed them for the lack of evidence which might have led to a conviction of Hodgkiss. He also noted that his and Clarke's advice on confidentiality to the RCP from 1896 had been misunderstood or misrepresented in a textbook of medical ethics, i.e. Saundby's book.[359]

Two weeks after the Hodgkiss trial, the Director of Public Prosecutions, Sir Charles Mathews (1850–1920), wrote to the solicitor of the British Medical Association, William Hempson, drawing attention to Justice Avory's comments and asking to make them widely known within the medical profession in order to correct the inaccuracy contained in Saundby's book regarding medical secrecy in cases involving a criminal offence (see above). Perhaps unexpectedly, Mathews received a firm response from Hempson in which he asked for permission to take the matter to the Central Ethical Committee (CEC) of the BMA. Moreover, Hempson

---

[358] Avory, cited in Cooke, *History of the Royal College*, vol. 3, p. 983. See also 'A Judge on Professional Secrecy', *The Lancet* 184 (1914), pp. 1430-1431.

[359] Avory, cited in Cooke, *History of the Royal College*, vol. 3, p. 983.

met with Mathews at Whitehall on 22 December 1914 to discuss the issue with him. While Mathews expressed his conviction that doctors had a higher duty to the state in aid of the suppression of crime than to their patients, Hempson was concerned that doctors might face litigation from patients if they disclosed in such cases, and he asked whether doctors would be protected against this by the state if they followed such a duty to report – something that Mathews could not commit to. Mathews told Hempson that the Lord Chief Justice, Lord Reading, also agreed with Avory's statement and had suggested to send a copy of it to all coroners in England and Wales for their attention.[360]

For the BMA's discussion of the issue, Hempson prepared in early January 1915 a memorandum in which he outlined the legal situation for medical confidentiality as he saw it. Whereas personal communications made to solicitors and barristers, as well as to ministers of religion under the confessional, were protected against disclosure, medical men could be forced by a judge in civil and criminal courts to answer questions pertaining to confidential information of their patients. Outside the court, Hempson advised, a medical practitioner who learned during treatment about a criminal offence that his patient had committed, was not obliged to report this. This was also his reading of Clarke

[360] Cf. Angus H. Ferguson, *Should a Doctor Tell? The Evolution of Medical Confidentiality in Britain* (Farnham and Burlington, Ashgate, 2013), pp. 43-45.

and Avory's 1896 advice to the Royal College of Physicians, even in the light of the latter's comments in the Hodgkiss trial. Hempson further pointed out that Avory's recent statement conflicted with Justice Hawkins' remarks on the issue in the *Kitson v. Playfair* case.[361] However, Hempson's interpretation differed from Mathews' position, which he summarised as follows:

> Sir Charles Mathews, the Public Prosecutor, is obviously interested in securing the assistance of the medical profession in the detection of crime. Viewing the matter generally he represents to me that they are citizens of the State who owe a higher duty to the State in detection of crime than they do to their patients. In support of Mr. Justice Avory's dictum he also contends that if a medical man in the course of his attendance upon and treatment of a patient becomes aware that a crime has been committed or indeed has reason confidently to believe that such is the case and the patient is believed by him to be in danger of death a duty rests upon such medical man incumbent upon him to discharge to place matters in train for a dying deposition being secured from the patient in question on the ground that otherwise the crime would go undetected and the person committing it would go scot free. Sir Charles denies that any greater

---

[361] 'The British Medical Association. Professional Secrecy. Notes and Memoranda by Mr. W. E. Hempson', SA/BMA/D170, BMA Archives, Wellcome Library, London.

protection in this connection is accorded to the medical profession than to any other members of the public.[362]

The BMA's Central Ethical Committee considered in a meeting on 8 January 1915 Hempson's information as well as a memorandum by Saundby, which defended his interpretation of Clarke and Avory's advice to the RCP and which had been approved by Aldridge and Jordan. Concerned about potential libel actions against medical practitioners if they reported without the patient's consent and the potential consequence that people would no longer see doctors in sensitive matters if their confidential information was not safe, the CEC arrived at three recommendations for the BMA Council: (1) that doctors must not disclose information without the patient's consent; (2) that, if the state was unable to protect doctors against legal actions following disclosure, the state had no right to demand from them to report information which they had obtained during treatment of patients; and (3) to openly discuss the matter in the *British Medical Journal* before sending the final resolution to the relevant state department. The last recommendation was in direct defiance of Sir Charles Mathews' wishes, who had asked Hempson to keep the matter out of the press. The Council adopted the CEC's recommendations on 27 January

---

[362] Ibid., pp. 3-4.

1915, even sharpening the second one by removing the conditional clause from it, so that it simply denied a right of the state to claiming patients' information from their doctors.[363]

Following further discussions between Mathews and Hempson, the issue was kept out of the press for the time being, but a deputation of the BMA met on 3 May 1915 with the Lord Chief Justice, the Attorney General, the Public Prosecutor and other legal authorities.[364] As a result of this meeting it was ascertained that 'it is desired by the Authorities that information should be given to them by medical men in attendance upon a woman suffering from the effects of abortion brought about by artificial intervention', but that there were three conditions limiting such reporting. The medical man had to be convinced, from his examination of the patient or from her communication to him, (1) that the abortion was due to artificial intervention, (2) that the intervention had been made by a third party, not by the woman herself, and (3) he had to be of the opinion that the woman was likely to die as a result of the intervention.[365]

These conditions represented a limitation of Avory's suggestion that doctors should also report cases of illegal abortion where the woman might well recover. Despite this

---

[363] Ferguson, *Should a Doctor Tell?*, pp. 45-48.

[364] Ibid., pp. 48-49.

[365] 'Extract from Supplementary Report of Council, Supplement, July 3, 1915. Medical Ethics, Professional Secrecy', SA/BMA/D167, BMA Archives, Wellcome Library, London.

clarification, the BMA Council adhered, however, to its position from January, and on 3 July 1915 issued a resolution stating that (1) 'a medical practitioner should not under any circumstances disclose voluntarily, without the patient's consent, information which he has obtained from that patient in the exercise of his professional duties' and that (2) 'the State has no right to claim that an obligation rests upon a medical practitioner to disclose voluntarily information which he has obtained in the exercise of professional duties'.[366]

Mathews had also contacted the Royal College of Physicians, asking its Censors' Board whether they agreed with Justice Avory's opinion. As it happened, a fellow of the RCP had been sitting on the grand jury of the Hodgkiss trial, so was familiar with the details of the case. He informed the Censors' Board that while Ellen Armstrong had been very ill, she had died unexpectedly. In a meeting with the Board on 26 January 1915, Mathews expressed his view that a medical practitioner was obliged to inform the police if he was convinced that a woman had had a criminal abortion and was likely to die from its effects, so that a statement could be taken from her which might be used as evidence in court. The Board's initial response was that they could not give an opinion, as Avory had not been aware of the fact that Armstrong's death was unexpected. However, after

[366] Ibid., *Minutes* 542 and 550.

further discussions, the RCP issued a resolution on the issue. It took the view that a medical practitioner was not entitled to disclose information without the woman's consent. However, it advised, in cases where the woman was seriously ill or dying after an illegal abortion, that he should urge her to make a formal statement that could be used as evidence against the abortionist. If she refused, he should not pursue the matter further and continue to treat her to the best of his ability. Before taking any action, the practitioner should seek medical and legal advice to ensure that the woman's statement was valid and to protect himself against subsequent litigation. If the woman died, he should refuse to fill in a death certificate and instead inform the coroner.[367]

The Royal College of Surgeons likewise rejected Avory's notion of a medical practitioner's duty to report criminal abortions. In a letter to Mathews, on 2 July 1915, it emphasised the high value of medical confidentiality for patients and the public. Unwilling to formulate specific rules, the RCS wanted to leave the matter to the individual practitioner's discretion in each case. The decision to keep secrecy or to report should rest on the practitioner's conscience and sense of duty to his patient and the state.[368] As an editorial

---

367 Cooke, *History of the Royal College*, vol. 3, pp. 984-985.
368 Ferguson, *Should a Doctor Tell?*, p. 50.

in the *Lancet* aptly summed up the medical profession's general position:

> The medical man is there to save the patient's life and to restore the patient to health if he can; not to aid the police by playing the detective. [...] If he once reveals his patient's secret, [...] he will destroy belief in his professional discretion [...] and any general adoption of his course of action would diminish or destroy all trust in his profession everywhere.[369]

The organised medical profession's advice to practitioners was thus quite clear: preservation of patient confidentiality and, through this, of the practitioner's reputation, came before any duty to the state to assist in detecting a criminal offence. While some practitioners might have chosen to report cases of illegal abortion to the police,[370] most would have followed the line of their professional bodies and reported only, with the woman's consent, if she was likely to die from the intervention, or indeed after her death. Keeping confidentiality, and not to report, matched public expectations about medical secrecy. For example, in 1930, such expectations were powerfully conveyed in a popular

---

[369] 'A Judge on Professional Secrecy' (Editorial), *The Lancet* 185 (1915), p. 28.

[370] See e.g. W. H. Willcox, 'Criminal Abortion and Professional Secrecy', ibid., pp. 97-98, who argued that an abortion should be reported to the authorities, also without patient consent, if there was 'conclusive objective evidence of criminal interference', as the medical practitioner's duty to the public and to himself would override his obligation of secrecy to the patient in such a case.

film entitled *Should a Doctor Tell?* in which a London consultant discovers that his son's fiancée is the same woman who has some time ago asked for his medical help when she had become pregnant in a relationship with a married man. Her child having meanwhile 'died', she implores the consultant: 'I want your silence. I don't plead with you as a father, I demand it of you as a Doctor!'[371]

Confidentiality in Venereal Diseases and in Court

While doctors' moral choice appears to have favoured confidentiality in abortion cases, the matter was more controversial in another situation. Having a patient with a venereal disease such as syphilis or gonorrhoea who was unwilling to take precautions, should a doctor then breach the patient's confidence and warn others of the risk of infection?

The debate over disclosure of venereal diseases needs to be seen in its contemporary legal context. On the one hand, medical practitioners in Britain were (and still are) obliged to give medical evidence in court, including confidential patient details, if required to do so by the judge. This so-called lack of medical privilege in court originated from a prece-

---

[371] *Should a Doctor Tell?*, a British Lion Production, dialogue by Edgar Wallace, directed by Manning Haynes [Press kit, London, 1930], British Film Institute.

dent in 1776, the trial in front of the House of Peers of Elizabeth Chudleigh (1720-1788), Duchess of Kingston, for bigamy. When asked by counsel for the prosecution about an earlier secret marriage of the Duchess, her surgeon and friend, Caesar Hawkins (1711-1786), had initially been unwilling to give evidence, raising the question whether it was consistent with his professional honour to disclose something that had come before him 'in a confidential trust' in his profession.[372] Lord Chief Justice Mansfield (William Murray, 1705-1793) replied that if 'a Surgeon was voluntarily to reveal these Secrets, to be sure he would be guilty of a Breach of Honour, and of great Indiscretion; but to give that Information in a Court of Justice, which by the Law of the Land he is bound to do, will never be imputed to him as any Indiscretion whatever'.[373] Caesar Hawkins subsequently testified, and the Duchess was found guilty.

The principle of Lord Mansfield's opinion, that there was no privilege for medical witnesses, was adopted by other English courts, developing into a common law rule.[374] This

---

[372] *The Trial of Elizabeth Duchess Dowager of Kingston for Bigamy, Before the Right Honourable House of Peers,* in Westminster-Hall, in Full Parliament...Published by Order of the House of Peers (London, Charles Bathurst, 1776), p. 119.

[373] Ibid., p. 120. See also Thomas Bayly Howell, *A Complete Collection of State Trials,* vol. 20 (London: Longman, Hurst, Rees etc., 1816), pp. 572-573.

[374] Angus H, Ferguson, 'The Lasting Legacy of a Bigamous Duchess: The Benchmark Precedent for Medical Confidentiality', *Social History of Medicine* 19 (2006), pp. 37-53; Danuta Mendelson, 'The Duchess of Kingston's Case, the Ruling of Lord Mansfield and Duty of Medical Confidentiality in Court', *International Journal of Law and Psychiatry* 35 (2012), pp. 480-489.

became particularly sensitive in divorce trials, when one party sought to establish through a medical witness that the other party had infected them with a venereal disease, in order to prove adultery and cruelty. For men seeking a divorce, proof of the wife's adultery was required, whereas women needed to prove their husband's cruelty as well as adultery to be granted a divorce.[375]

On the other hand, English VD policy in the late nineteenth and early twentieth century followed a 'voluntarist' approach which counted on free access to *confidential* diagnosis and therapy rather than notification to health authorities and compulsory treatment. A specific historical background to this rather liberal approach was the repeal, in 1886, of the Contagious Diseases Acts of the 1860s, which had provided for the compulsory medical inspection and treatment of female prostitutes in garrison and naval towns, and had attracted much criticism by the early women's movement and the churches as consolidating 'vice'.[376] At-

---

375 Maehle, *Contesting Medical Confidentiality*, pp. 29-33; Ferguson, *Should a Doctor Tell?*, p. 61.

376 Lesley A. Hall, 'Venereal Diseases and Society in Britain, from the Contagious Diseases Acts to the National Health Service', in Roger Davidson and Lesley A. Hall (eds), *Sex, Sin and Suffering: Venereal Disease in European Society since 1870* (London, Routledge, 2001), pp. 120-136; Roger Davidson and Lutz D. H. Sauerteig, 'Law, Medicine and Morality: A Comparative View of Twentieth-Century Sexually Transmitted Disease Controls', in John Woodward and Robert Jütte (eds), *Coping with Sickness: Medicine, Law and Human Rights – Historical Perspectives* (Sheffield, EAHMH Publications, 2000), pp. 127-147.

tempts in the 1880s and 1890s to introduce compulsory notification of venereal diseases through legal powers of local authorities and provisions of the Infectious Diseases (Notification) Act of 1889 failed, not least because of the opposition of doctors who argued that such reporting of VD would undermine the confidential nature of the relationship to their patients. VD patients would be driven away from qualified medical practitioners into the hands of unscrupulous quacks, so notification would be counterproductive.[377]

The ethical question remained, however, whether a medical practitioner should warn known contact persons who might be at risk of infection from his patient. A typical scenario was that of a syphilitic fiancé who did not want his future wife to know about his condition, or that of a husband who had contracted a sexually transmitted disease in an extramarital affair and refused to tell his wife about it. Robert Saundby's advice in his *Medical Ethics* (1907) was to try to dissuade the ill fiancé from his marriage plans and to urge VD patients to take all necessary precautions for preventing infection. However, the disease was not meant to be disclosed to contact persons without the patient's consent.[378] Saundby's position reflected a general reluctance of medical practitioners to go beyond appealing to the VD patient's

[377] Graham Mooney, 'Public Health and Private Practice: The Contested Development of Compulsory Infectious Disease Notification in Late-Nineteenth-Century Britain', *Bulletin of the History of Medicine* 73 (1999), pp. 238-267.
[378] Saundby, *Medical Ethics*, pp. 68, 116.

conscience. Yet, there were opposing voices as well. Campbell Williams, a fellow of the Royal College of Surgeons, regretted in a lecture before the Harveian Society, published in the *Lancet* in 1906, that syphilis and gonorrhoea did not belong to the list of notifiable diseases. In light of the damage that venereal disease might cause to the wife of an infected husband, he thought the medical practitioner should warn her, even if the disclosure might lead to divorce. However, even Williams stuck to the rule not to inform the wife about the nature of the illness if she was already infected. In this case, he claimed, ignorance was 'bliss'. If a household servant, cook, or nursemaid had contracted syphilis or gonorrhoea, the doctor should urge them to leave their job by threatening exposure, or, if necessary, disclose their illness to their employer.[379] Another fellow of the Royal College of Surgeons, Hunterian Professor J. Howell Evans, made a similar point in an address to the London Medico-Legal Society in 1908, arguing that if the employer had paid the medical attendant he was entitled to receive correct information about the servant's illness.[380]

There was, however, the risk that VD patients would sue their doctor for libel if he disclosed their illness to their employer without consent. A. G. Bateman, the secretary of the

---

[379] Campbell Williams, 'The Ethics of the Medical Profession in relation to Syphilis and Gonorrhoea', *The Lancet* 167 (1906), pp. 361-363.
[380] J. Howell Evans, 'The Medico-Legal Significance of Gonorrhoea', *Transactions of the Medico-Legal Society* 5 (1907/8), p. 157.

Medical Defence Union, gave examples of such cases. In one instance, a London fireman sued (unsuccessfully) the medical officer of the fire brigade for libel because the latter had reported the man's infection with venereal disease to his employer, which led to the man's dismissal. In another case a Leeds doctor was sued by the patient, a barmaid, as he had communicated her diagnosis to her employer, the housekeeper and her presumed husband as well as a fellow barmaid. While the court condoned the first three disclosures, it awarded damages of £75 due to the fourth communication.[381] By the early 1930s, doctors were explicitly advised against disclosures of VD without the patient's consent. As London consultant Francis G. Crookshank (1873–1933), a fellow of the Royal College of Physicians, wrote in a handbook chapter on the medico-legal aspects of venereal diseases in 1931:

> An employer has no sort of claim to obtain from a doctor attending an employee information as to the nature of a malady from which the latter may be suffering, without his express consent: in no case does payment of the doctor's fee, or a promise, express or implied, to pay the fee, give any shadow of right to such information [...].[382]

---

[381] A. G. Bateman, 'Professional Secrecy and Privileged Communications', *Transactions of the Medico-Legal Society* 2 (1904/5), pp. 57-59.

[382] F. G. Crookshank, 'The Medico-Legal Relations of Venereal Disease', in L. W. Harrison (ed.), *The Diagnosis and Treatment of Venereal Disease in General Practice*, 4th edn (London, Humphrey Milford, Oxford University Press, 1931), pp. 452-506, on p. 478.

Regarding the scenario between husband and wife, Crookshank was equally clear that neither of them had a right to the information without the other's consent:

> A husband has no sort of claim to obtain from a doctor, without his wife's consent, knowledge of a malady from which she may be suffering; and what is for the wife is also, in this respect, for the husband.[383]

By the time Crookshank was writing, the issue of disclosure of venereal diseases had been tested in two much-publicised divorce trials. During the First World War, concerns about an increase of venereal infections had led to official steps against the spread of VD. Under the Public Health (Venereal Disease) Regulations of 1916, the Local Government Board introduced a system of VD treatment centres, which offered confidential and free diagnosis and therapy. By the end of 1920, 185 such centres had been established in England and Wales.[384] Serious concerns arose, however, when doctors working for these confidential centres were called as witnesses in divorce proceedings and required by the judge to give evidence on their patient's illness. In one such trial, *Garner v. Garner* (1920), the doctor, Salomon Kadinski of the Westminster Hospital, protested against the request to testify on behalf of the wife who claimed to have been infected by her adulterous husband. The judge, Justice

383 Ibid.
384 Davidson and Sauerteig, 'Law, Medicine and Morality', p. 131.

Henry Alfred McCardie (1869–1933), however, rejected this protest, stating that there were 'even higher considerations' than the position of medical men, and Kadinski subsequently confirmed that she suffered from syphilis.[385] In another case, *Needham v. Needham* (1921), Dr John Elliott (1861–1921) of the VD clinic in Chester was subpoenaed to testify to the husband's claim that his wife had contracted gonorrhoea in an adulterous relationship. Encouraged by the Ministry of Heath, which intended to make this a test case for confidentiality in the VD treatment scheme, Elliott initially refused to give evidence, referring to the authority of the 1916 Regulations on VD. However, the judge, Justice Horridge, regarded them as insufficient to override a doctor's duty to give evidence in a court of law. Facing the prospect of a six-month prison sentence for contempt of court, Elliott gave in and testified.[386]

These and similar cases renewed in the 1920s the debate over confidentiality in venereal diseases.

---

[385] 'Law Report, Jan. 13', *The Times*, January 14, 1920, p. 5; 'Medical Evidence in Divorce. Effect on Treatment Schemes. Value of Secrecy', *The Times*, January 15, 1920; Digby Cotes-Preedy, 'Judges and Medical Privilege', *The Times*, January 15, 1920, p. 5; 'The Privacy of Venereal Clinics', *The Lancet* 195 (1920), p. 163; D. Harcourt Kitchin, *Law for the Medical Practitioner* (London, Eyre & Spottiswoode Ltd., 1941), pp. 160-161; Ferguson, *Should a Doctor Tell?*, pp. 61-63.

[386] 'A Doctor's Claim to Privilege. Needham v. Needham and Bennett', *The Times*, June 10, 1921, p. 4; 'Dr. John Elliott', *The Times*, December 20, 1921; Ferguson, *Should a Doctor Tell?*, pp. 71-77.

In contrast to the issue of medical secrecy in abortion cases, the British Medical Association was divided in its opinion.[387] When the BMA's solicitor Hempson, during a speech to its Annual Representative Meeting (ARM) 1920 in Cambridge, used the hypothetical example of the syphilitic fiancé, asking whether the bride's father should be informed about the condition of his future son-in-law, he received shouts of 'Yes!' as well as 'No!' from the audience. The ARM of this year passed a resolution that doctors must not disclose confidential information without the patient's consent, accepting, however, the exception that such information had to be given when demanded by a judge in a court of law. The ARM furthermore tasked the BMA Council 'to consider the extent to which, and the ways in which, the Association is prepared to support its Members in maintaining professional secrecy'. The BMA's Central Ethical Committee, having discussed professional secrecy in a special sub-committee, recommended to the Council to adopt the policy that if a medical practitioner refused to divulge information in court or to report an infectious disease which was notifiable by law, he could not expect the BMA to support him. In other situations of 'encroachment' on confidentiality, however, e.g. in attempts to compel doctors to act as

[387] For more detailed accounts of the BMA's views on issues of medical confidentiality, see Andrew A. G. Morrice, '"Should the doctor tell?" Medical secrecy in early twentieth-century Britain', in Steve Sturdy (ed.), *Medicine, Health and the Public Sphere in Britain, 1600-2000* (London and New York, Routledge, 2002), pp. 60-82; Ferguson, *Should a Doctor Tell?*, pp. 79-109.

informants for the detection of abortions, the BMA might support the medical practitioner.[388]

The Council put the recommended policy to the BMA's ARM meeting of 1921 in Newcastle. However, by that time the trial of *Needham v. Needham*, with Justice Horridge forcing Dr Elliott to testify despite his protest, had radicalised delegates' opinions on the matter. The ARM rejected the proposed policy and adopted instead the resolution that 'the Association use all its power to support a member of the British Medical Association who refuses to divulge, without the patient's consent, information obtained in the exercise of his professional duties, except where it is already provided by Act of Parliament that he must do so'.[389]

A dichotomy was thus revealed within the British Medical Association on the question of whether a medical practitioner had to disclose patient information in legal proceedings, with the BMA basis wanting the Association to give full, including financial, support to doctors who found themselves in a situation like Elliott, whereas the Central Ethical Committee wished to preserve the status quo, i.e.

---

[388] 'Extract from BMA Council Agenda of February 16, 1921', SA/BMA/D168, BMA Archives, Wellcome Library, London; Ferguson, *Should a Doctor Tell?*, pp. 80-83.

[389] 'Proceedings of Council, March 8th, 1922, as to Question of Professional Secrecy', British Medical Association, Central Ethical Committee, Meeting March 31st, 1922, SA/BMA/D168, BMA Archives, Wellcome Library, London; Ferguson, *Should a Doctor Tell?*, p. 84.

was in principle willing to accept a doctor's duty to give evidence in a court of law. After the Newcastle resolution, the CEC reconsidered the issue and reported in a special meeting of Council on 8 March 1922. As the CEC chairman, Dr Reginald Langdon Down (1866–1955), summed up the committee's position, the resolution of the Newcastle meeting should not encourage BMA members to take now a generally defiant attitude in courts of law and to refuse giving evidence without good reason. The only acceptable reason to claim medical privilege in court was, in his opinion, *public* interest. While the patient's interest in confidentiality was important, it had in his view been exaggerated from its notion in the Hippocratic Oath, and patients should not be able to force doctors to do something contrary to the general will. In his opinion 'the judge, sitting between the parties, was best able to say whether the doctor's evidence should be given or not'. Langdon Down admitted, however, that, as judges were 'not infallible', it would be necessary to provide for cases in which a judge 'misunderstood' his function. He hoped that an agreed report could be taken to the next Annual Representative Meeting for discussion.[390]

The BMA Council members, however, were dissatisfied with Langdon Down's proposal. In particular they demanded more exact formulations of 'the conditions under which, the extent to which, and the ways in which' the BMA

[390] 'Proceedings of Council, March 8th, 1922', p. 1.

would support a medical practitioner who refused to give evidence in court, and referred the matter back to the CEC for this purpose. Following a suggestion of Langdon Down, several Council members were delegated to assist in this task, reflecting the high-profile status that the issue of medical confidentiality had reached in the BMA.[391]

The augmented CEC sub-committee on professional secrecy discussed the problem in detail, also considering underlying principles, in two meetings in March and April 1922. Among others, Langdon Down's points about the public interest criterion and about judges being best placed to decide whether medical evidence was necessary, were challenged by two Council members: Dr Ernest Fothergill put emphasis on the patient's interest as the factor that would morally justify a medical man to refuse giving evidence in court; and Dr Guy Dain warned that some judges might compel the medical evidence out of convenience, as it might speed up a trial, not considering the potential damage to public confidence in doctors' secrecy.[392] BMA solicitor Hempson had prepared a memorandum, in which he drew attention to another problem. If a patient sued a medical practitioner for malpractice, and had also been treated by a few other doctors, the plaintiff's side was likely to call only those doctors as witnesses who might support their

---

[391] Ibid., p. 2. See also Ferguson, *Should a Doctor Tell?*, pp. 90-93.

[392] Ferguson, *Should a Doctor Tell?*, pp. 95, 97.

case, not those who might exonerate the accused practitioner. If the defendant's side then called the latter doctors, the patient would probably refuse consent to them testifying. If they then refused to give evidence to protect patient confidentiality, they might harm through this their accused colleague. How would the BMA view their refusal?[393] A practical proposal by Council member Arnold Lyndon, that the BMA should only support members who in the Council's and CEC's opinion were justified in their refusal to give evidence, was accepted, as it would have made the BMA leadership the arbiter and protected the BMA's financial resources.[394]

Put to the ARM meeting of 1922, in Glasgow, by Langdon Down, Lyndon's proposal was also accepted there. Moreover, Langdon Down achieved a more moderate stance of the BMA by having a further proposal accepted saying that 'the proper preservation of professional secrecy necessitates a measure of special consideration being recognised for medical witnesses in courts of law above and beyond what is accorded to the ordinary witness'.

It was also agreed that patient consent to disclosure was essential.[395]

---

393 'Professional Secrecy. Notes and Memoranda by the Solicitor, 4th April 1922', SA/BMA/D170, BMA Archives, Wellcome Library, London.
394 Ferguson, *Should a Doctor Tell?*, pp. 98-99.
395 Ibid., p. 107.

Such a moderate move towards a medical privilege in court relied on a measure of co-operation of the judiciary. This co-operation, however, was not forthcoming; to the contrary, a privilege for medical witnesses was firmly resisted by the judiciary. In particular, the Lord Chancellor, Viscount Birkenhead (Frederick Edwin Smith, 1872–1930), had written in late 1921 an essay against a medical privilege, which he distributed to all judges and Lords of Appeal and which was published in the following year. His key argument was that allowing an exception for medical confidentiality would obstruct judges in their work and thus hinder the administration of justice. As Birkenhead argued, 'to establish a class who may at their will assist or obstruct the judges in their work would be a retrograde step not justified by any argument which has been brought forward'.[396] Facing such formidable opposition, the BMA Council decided in early 1923 to postpone the matter for six months, and in September of that year, indefinitely.[397]

The uncompromising position of judges on the question of a medical privilege was demonstrated again by Justice McCardie in a Birmingham divorce trial in 1927. He compelled medical evidence on the husband's alleged venereal disease regardless of the governmental guarantee of confidentiality in the VD treatment centres and despite the fact

---

[396] Viscount Birkenhead, *Points of View* (London, Hodder and Stoughton Limited, 1922), vol. 1, p. 75.
[397] Ferguson, *Should a Doctor Tell?*, p.109.

that the medical staff concerned had protested against the demand to disclose.[398] McCardie subsequently justified his position in an address to the Medico-Legal Society. As the London correspondent of the *Journal of the American Medical Association* reported about this speech:

> There were two aspects of the question [of medical secrecy], each of which was vital. There was the physician who said, 'Health, health, health, and break down the legal obstacles that prevent the gain of health.' Yes, but there was another point of view – and there was not a lawyer whose heart was not stirred – and that was 'Truth, truth, truth; open the shutters and let in the light of truth. Truth lay at the root of criminal justice.'[399]

Efforts of the Ministry of Health to achieve a protection of medical secrecy only in civil cases, such as divorce proceedings, likewise failed due to the resistance of the judiciary. A private member's bill to permit a medical privilege in court for VD cases, introduced into Parliament in 1927 by the MP and dermatologist Ernest Gordon Graham-Little (1867–1950), failed, as did his second attempt in 1936-37 with a bill for a wider medical privilege.[400]

---

[398] 'Professional Secrecy of Doctors. Mr Justice McCardie on Duty to Court', *The Times*, July 19, 1927, p. 11; E. Graham Little, 'Medical Privilege. Doctors and the Courts', *The Times*, November 14, 1927, p. 10; Ferguson, *Should a Doctor Tell?*, pp. 130-131.

[399] 'Foreign Letters: London: Law and Medicine', *Journal of the American Medical Association* 90 (1928), p. 629.

[400] See Ferguson, *Should a Doctor Tell?*, pp. 138-153.

While doctors were thus left with little or no choice when they were demanded to testify in court regarding venereal diseases or other sensitive conditions of their patients, they still could exercise discretion in daily practice whether they felt morally obliged to disclose a particular VD case. For example, writing in 1921 W. G. Aitchison Robertson, a lecturer in medical jurisprudence at Edinburgh University, argued that in the situation of the syphilitic fiancé, who wants to keep his illness secret, the doctor should inform the father-in-law. The breach of confidentiality would occur here in the interest of others, and it was unconceivable that a court would find the doctor culpable in such a case.[401] In contrast to Robertson, Hugh Woods, the secretary of the London and Counties Medical Protection Society, advised in 1924 that it was not a doctor's duty to disclose the fiancé's syphilis in this situation. If it was, he asked sarcastically, why not also reveal that he was a drunkard or had other objectionable characteristics?[402]

The discretion of the doctor in making a decision in such cases was also recognised from a legal perspective. Lord Riddell (George Allardice Riddell, 1865–1934), suggested in 1927, in a lecture for the Medico-Legal Society, that doctors

[401] W. G. Aitchison Robertson, *Medical Conduct and Practice: A Guide to the Ethics of Medicine* (London, A. & C. Black, 1921), p. 134.

[402] Hugh Woods, 'Medical Secrecy', *The Lancet* 203 (1924), p. 853; also in *The Conduct of Medical Practice*, ed. by the Editor of *The Lancet* and Expert Collaborators (London, *The Lancet*, 1927), pp. 78-83.

might be able to claim a right to disclose on the basis of a 'public duty to prevent wrongful acts'. As Riddle argued,

> The terrible consequences to innocent persons of secrecy in the hypothetical cases of the syphilitic husband or wife, the diseased fiancé, the syphilitic cook or nurse [...] are matters deeply concerning the public welfare. Disclosure to avoid such consequences is justifiable and perhaps obligatory on both legal and ethical grounds.[403]

However, he wanted to leave the final decision to disclose to the personal conscience of the individual medical practitioner in each case. Similarly Crookshank, in the above-mentioned handbook article, advised the practitioner to explain the position to the patient and then to follow his personal judgement and conscience. The health and happiness of innocent persons should not be risked through the doctor's timidity, though he should consult his medical defence society as he might face legal action from the patient if he decided to warn contacts.[404]

Doctors were thus left in the end with their personal ethical judgement about keeping confidentiality in VD cases outside court. They risked being sued if they disclosed without the patient's consent. However, as London barrister D. Harcourt Kitchin suggested in his handbook on medical law in 1941, if the disclosure was made to protect the health of

---

[403] Lord Riddell, *Medico-Legal Problems* (London, H. K. Lewis & Co., 1929), p. 58.

[404] Crookshank, 'Medico-Legal Relations', pp. 460, 464

others, such as wife, fiancée, or fellow workers, 'the court might take the view that a moral duty to disclose constituted a good defence'.[405]

Conclusions

As these examples show, a number of different factors could influence the moral choices of nineteenth-century medical practitioners. In the issue of reporting illegal abortions to the authorities, a medical practitioner's attitude towards the state and the law might have been important. However, of paramount concern for doctors were the health and trust of the women who sought his help when serious complications occurred after the intervention. The British medical professional organisations unanimously protected this priority, making it clear that the state had no claim to this confidential patient information (except as evidence in a court of law), so that it was the individual practitioner's decision to report a case of criminal abortion, with the patient's consent, or to remain silent.

In the question of warning contacts of patients suffering from a venereal disease, doctors were more inclined to disregard confidentiality in the interest of 'innocent' others, especially marital partners. Disclosure with the patient's consent was the preferred option, but where consent was

[405] Kitchin, *Law for the Medical Practitioner*, p. 282.

refused, practitioners faced the risk of legal action by the patient if they warned contact persons regardless. Remaining silent in this situation may therefore have had less to do with a commitment to patient confidentiality than with the fear of legal consequences. A dual loyalty conflict, between the interest of the patient and the interest of the state, existed also for medical practitioners when subpoenaed as witnesses in court. Following the judge's order and testifying against the patient's will could lead to litigation from the patient; but in refusing to give evidence, in the interest of the patient, the medical witness risked imprisonment for contempt of court. Overall, nineteenth-century doctors thus had to navigate complex situations in which their decisions were influenced by their personal moral views and sense of professional honour, the position taken by their professional organisations, and social as well as legal pressures.

Select Bibliography

- Francis Bacon, *The Advancement of Learning*, ed. by Michael Kiernan (Oxford, Clarendon Press, 2000)
- Robert Baker, *Before Bioethics: A History of American Medical Ethics from the Colonial Period to the Bioethics Revolution* (New York, Oxford University Press, 2013)
- Robert Baker, Dorothy Porter and Roy Porter (eds), *The Codification of Medical Morality*, vol. 1: *Medical Ethics and Etiquette in the Eighteenth Century* (Dordrecht, Kluwer Academic Publishers, 1993)
- Robert Baker (ed.), *The Codification of Medical Morality*, vol. 2: *Anglo-American Medical Ethics and Medical Jurisprudence in the Nineteenth Century* (Dordrecht, Kluwer Academic Publishers, 1995)
- Robert Baker and Laurence B. McCullough (eds), *The Cambridge World History of Medical Ethics* (New York, Cambridge University Press, 2009)
- Norman Batesby, *Medical Chaos and Crime* (London and New York, Mitchell Kennerley, 1910)
- Jeffrey Lionel Berlant, *Profession and Monopoly: A Study of Medicine in the United States and Great Britain* (Berkeley, University of California Press, 1975)
- Jochen Binder, *Zwischen Standesrecht und Marktwirtschaft: Ärztliche Werbung zu Beginn des 20. Jahrhunderts im*

deutsch-englischen Vergleich (Frankfurt/M., Peter Lang, 2000)

- Viscount Birkenhead, *Points of View* (London, Hodder and Stoughton Limited, 1922)
- James Blundell, *The Principles and Practice of Obstetricy, to which are added, Notes and Illustrations, by Thomas Castle* (Washington, Duff Green, 1834)
- Rob Boddice, *The Science of Sympathy: Morality, Evolution, and Victorian Civilization* (Urbana, University of Illinois Press, 2016)
- Howard Brody, Zahra Meghani and Kimberly Greenwald (eds), *Michael Ryan's Writings on Medical Ethics* (Dordrecht, Springer, 2010)
- Barbara Brookes, *Abortion in England, 1900-1967* (London, Croom Helm, 1988)
- Michael Brown, *Performing medicine: Medical culture and identity in provincial England, c. 1760-1850* (Manchester and New York, Manchester University Press, 2011)
- Robert Brudenell Carter, *Doctors and Their Work or Medicine, Quackery, and Disease* (London, Smith, Elder, & Co., 1903)
- Ian A. Burney, *Bodies of Evidence: Medicine and the Politics of the English Inquest 1830-1926* (Baltimore and London, Johns Hopkins University Press, 2000)
- Daniel Callahan, *In Search of the Good: A Life in Bioethics* (Cambridge, Mass. and London, MIT Press, 2012)

- Carl Capellmann, *Pastoral Medicine*, transl. by William Dassel (New York and Cincinnati, Fr. Pustet, 1879)
- M. Cooke, *A History of the Royal College of Physicians of London*, vol. 3 (Oxford, Clarendon Press, 1972)
- Roger Cooter and John Pickstone (eds), *Companion to Medicine in the Twentieth Century* (London and New York, Routledge, 2003)
- Roger Cooter with Claudia Stein, *Writing History in the Age of Biomedicine* (New Haven and London, Yale University Press, 2013)
- Charles Coppens, *Moral Principles and Medical Practice: The Basis of Medical Jurisprudence* (New York, Cincinnati and Chicago, Benziger Brothers, 1897)
- Ann Dally, *Fantasy Surgery, 1880-1930: with special reference to Sir William Arbuthnot Lane* (Amsterdam and Atlanta, Rodopi, 1996)
- Ann Dally, *Women under the Knife: A History of Surgery* (Edison, NJ, Castle Books, 2006)
- Roger Davidson and Lesley A. Hall (eds), *Sex, Sin and Suffering: Venereal Disease in European Society since 1870* (London, Routledge, 2001)
- Adrian J. Desmond, *The Politics of Evolution: Morphology, Medicine and Reform* (Chicago, University of Chicago Press, 1989)
- Anne Digby, *Making a Medical Living: Doctors and Patients in the English Market for Medicine, 1720-1911* (Cambridge, Cambridge University Press, 1994)

- Anne Digby, *The Evolution of General Practice 1850-1948* (Oxford and New York, Oxford University Press, 1999)
- Ian Dowbiggin, *A Concise History of Euthanasia: Life, Death, God, and Medicine* (Lanham, Rowan & Littlefield Publishers, 2005)
- John J. Elwell, *A Medico-Legal Treatise on Malpractice and Medical Evidence, Comprising the Elements of Medical Jurisprudence* (New York, John S. Voorhies, 1860)
- Ruth R. Faden and Tom L. Beauchamp in collaboration with Nancy M. P. King, *A History and Theory of Informed Consent* (New York and Oxford, Oxford University Press, 1986)
- Phil Fennel, *Treatment without Consent: Law, psychiatry and the treatment of mentally disordered people since 1845* (London and New York, Routledge, 1996)
- Angus H. Ferguson, *Should a Doctor Tell? The Evolution of Medical Confidentiality in Britain* (Farnham and Burlington, Ashgate, 2013)
- Roger French and Andrew Wear (eds), *British Medicine in an Age of Reform* (London, Routledge, 1991)
- Thomas Gisborne, *An Enquiry into the Duties of Men in the Higher and Middle Classes of Society in Great Britain, Resulting from their Respective Stations, Professions, and Employments*, 3rd edn (London, B. and J. White, 1795)
- David Gladstone (ed.), *Regulating Doctors* (London, Institute for the Study of Civil Society, 2000)
- John Gregory, *Lectures on the Duties and Qualifications of a Physician* (London, W. Strahan and T. Cadell, 1772)

- Lisbeth Haakonssen, *Medicine and Morals in the Enlightenment: John Gregory, Thomas Percival and Benjamin Rush* (Amsterdam, Rodopi, 1997)
- L. W. Harrison (ed.), *The Diagnosis and Treatment of Venereal Disease in General Practice*, 4th edn (London, Humphrey Milford, Oxford University Press, 1931)
- Thomas Bayly Howell, *A Complete Collection of State Trials*, vol. 20 (London, Longman, Hurst, Rees etc, 1816)
- Donald Irvine, *The Doctors' Tale: Professionalism and Public Trust* (Abingdon, Radcliffe Medical Press, 2003)
- Pat Jalland, *Death in the Victorian Family* (Oxford, Oxford University Press, 1996)
- Albert R. Jonsen, *The Birth of Bioethics* (New York and Oxford, Oxford University Press, 1998)
- Jay Katz, *The Silent World of Doctor and Patient* (New York, The Free Press, 1986)
- David F. Kelly, *The Emergence of Catholic Medical Ethics in North America: An Historical-Methodological-Bibliographical Study* (New York and Toronto, Edwin Mellen Press, 1979)
- N. D. A. Kemp, *'Merciful release'. The history of the British euthanasia movement* (Manchester and New York, Manchester University Press, 2002)
- John Keown, *Abortion, doctors and the law: Some aspects of the legal regulation of abortion in England from 1803 to 1982* (Cambridge, Cambridge University Press, 2002)

- D. Harcourt Kitchin, *Law for the Medical Practitioner* (London, Eyre & Spottiswoode Ltd., 1941)
- Susan C. Lawrence, *Charitable Knowledge: Hospital Pupils and Practitioners in Eighteenth-Century London* (New York, Cambridge University Press, 1996)
- Chauncey D. Leake (ed.), *Percival's Medical Ethics* (Huntington, NY, Robert E. Krieger Publishing Company, 1975)
- Andreas-Holger Maehle, *Contesting Medical Confidentiality: Origins of the Debate in the United States, Britain, and Germany* (Chicago and London, University of Chicago Press, 2016)
- Andreas-Holger Maehle, *Doctors, Honour and the Law: Medical Ethics in Imperial Germany* (Basingstoke, Palgrave Macmillan, 2009)
- Andreas-Holger Maehle and Johanna Geyer-Kordesch (eds), *Historical and Philosophical Perspectives on Biomedical Ethics: From Paternalism to Autonomy?* (Aldershot, Ashgate, 2002)
- Laurence B. McCullough, *John Gregory and the Invention of Professional Medical Ethics and the Profession of Medicine* (Dordrecht, Kluwer Academic Publishers, 1998)
- Laurence B. McCullough, *John Gregory's Writings on Medical Ethics and Philosophy of Medicine* (Dordrecht, Kluwer Academic Publishers, 1998)
- Angus McLaren, *Birth Control in Nineteenth-Century England* (New York, Holmes & Meier Publishers, 1978)

- Steven H. Miles, *The Hippocratic Oath and the Ethics of Medicine* (New York, Oxford University Press, 2004)
- Ornella Moscucci, *The Science of Woman: Gynaecology and Gender in England, 1800-1929* (Cambridge, New York and Melbourne, Cambridge University Press, 1993)
- Thomas Percival, *Medical Ethics* (Oxford 1849, Reprint Leopold Classic Library)
- E. H. Pitcairn (ed.), *Unwritten Laws and Ideals of Active Careers* (London, Smith, Elder, & Co, 1899)
- Walter F. Pratt, *Privacy in Britain* (Lewisburg, Bucknell University Press, and London, Associated University Presses, 1979)
- Kim Price, *Medical Negligence in Victorian Britain: The Crisis of Care under the English Poor Law, c. 1834-1900* (London, Bloomsbury Academic, 2015)
- Walter Pyke-Lees, *Centenary of the General Medical Council 1858-1958: The History and Present Work of the Council* (London, William Clowes & Sons, [1958])
- Francis H. Rambotham, *The Principles and Practice of Obstetric Medicine and Surgery, in Reference to the Process of Parturition.* A New Edition, from the Enlarged and Revised London Edition (Philadelphia, Lea & Blanchard, 1845)
- Jonathan Reinarz and Rebecca Wynter (eds), *Complaints, Controversies and Grievances in Medicine: Historical and social science perspectives* (London and New York, Routledge, 2015)

- Lord Riddell, *Medico-Legal Problems* (London, H. K. Lewis & Co., 1929)
- W. G. Aitchison Robertson, *Medical Conduct and Practice: A Guide to the Ethics of Medicine* (London, A. & C. Black, 1921)
- David J. Rothman, *Strangers at the Bedside: A History of How Law and Bioethics Transformed Medical Decision Making* (BasicBooks USA, 1991)
- Nicolaas A. Rupke (ed.), *Vivisection in Historical Perspective* (London, Routledge, 1990)
- William Sanderson and E. B. A. Rayner, *An Introduction to the Law and Tradition of Medical Practice* (London, H. K. Lewis & Co., 1926)
- Robert Saundby, *Medical Ethics: A Guide to Professional Conduct*, 2nd edn (London, Charles Griffin & Company, 1907)
- Thomas Schlich and Christopher Crenner (eds), *Technological Change in Modern Surgery: Historical Perspectives on Innovation* (Rochester, NY, University of Rochester Press, 2017)
- Andrew Scull, *Hysteria: The Biography* (Oxford and New York, Oxford University Press, 2009)
- Mark William Skippen, *Obstetric practice and cephalopelvic disproportion in Glasgow between 1840 and 1900* (PhD thesis, University of Glasgow, 2009)

- Russell G. Smith, *Medical Discipline: The Professional Conduct Jurisdiction of the General Medical Council, 1858-1990* (Oxford, Clarendon Press, 1994)
- Margaret Stacey, *Regulating British Medicine: The General Medical Council* (Chichester, John Wiley & Sons, 1992)
- Meinolfus Strätling, *Die Begründung der neuzeitlichen Medizinethik in Praxis, Lehre und Forschung: John Gregory (1724-1773) und seine Lectures on the Duties and Qualifications of a Physician* (Frankfurt/Main, Peter Lang, 1998)
- Steve Sturdy (ed.), *Medicine, Health and the Public Sphere in Britain, 1600-2000* (London and New York, Routledge, 2002)
- Jukes Styrap, *A Code of Medical Ethics: With Remarks on the Duties of Practitioners to their Patients, and the Obligations of Patients to their Medical Advisers: also on the Duties of the Profession to the Public, and the Obligations of the Public to the Faculty* (London, J. & A. Churchill, 1878)
- Lionel A. Tollemache, *Stones of Stumbling* (London, Hodgson & Son, 1884)
- Robert M. Veatch, *Disrupted Dialogue: Medical Ethics and the Collapse of Physician-Humanist Communication (1770-1980)* (New York, Oxford University Press, 2005)
- Ivan Waddington, *The Medical Profession in the Industrial Revolution* (Dublin, Gill and Macmillan, 1984)
- Andrew Wear, Johanna Geyer-Kordesch and Roger French (eds), *Doctors and Ethics: The Earlier Historical Setting of Professional Ethics* (Amsterdam, Rodopi, 1993)

- Adrian Wilson, *Ritual and Conflict: The Social Relations of Childbirth in Early Modern England* (Farnham and Burlington, Ashgate, 2013)
- Duncan Wilson, *The Making of British Bioethics* (Manchester, Manchester University Press, 2014)
- Jacqueline H. Wolf, *Cesarean Section: An American History of Risk, Technology, and Consequence* (Baltimore, Johns Hopkins University Press, 2018)
- John Woodward and Robert Jütte (eds), *Coping with Sickness: Medicine, Law and Human Rights – Historical Perspectives* (Sheffield, EAHMH Publications, 2000)

Acknowledgements

I am grateful for the participants' feedback that I received when presenting parts of this book at conferences of the European Association for the History of Medicine and Health (Bucharest 2017), the Society for the Social History of Medicine (Liverpool 2018) and the American Association for the History of Medicine (Columbus/Ohio 2019) and at several workshops of Durham University's Centre for the History of Medicine & Disease and Department of Philosophy (2017-19). I would also like to thank Rob Johnson of Ockham Publishing for his initial suggestion to write on the history of medical ethics for a wide readership and his encouragement throughout the process. Moreover, I am grateful to Sarah Hembrow of Ockham Publishing for her careful editorial work. Last but not least, thanks to my wife Jillian and my daughter Sophie for their comments from a legal perspective.

Made in United States
North Haven, CT
10 November 2026

22079941R00120